Dyslexia Defined

Macdonald Critchley

and

Eileen A. Critchley

WILLIAM HEINEMANN MEDICAL BOOKS LTD
London

H P J

First published 1978

© M. Critchley and E. A. Critchley 1978

ISBN 0 433 06704 7

Printed and bound in Great Britain
by R. J. Acford Ltd., Chichester, Sussex

Contents

Introduction

There is a superabundance of books about developmental dyslexia and other reading difficulties, but we feel there is still room for a volume which is addressed to enquiring parents and teachers and which deals with the fundamental problems of dyslectic children. It was not our intention to "write down", nor to use too many medical terms, nor to compete with the multitude of publications which describe methods of teaching a child to read. Here and there the reader will observe some overlap. This is deliberate, for it permits each chapter to be read in isolation, and not necessarily sequentially with the book as a whole.

The subject of developmental dyslexia should intrigue any thoughtful person who wonders why it is that Man, alone among the animal species, is endowed with the mysterious gift of language; and that, in favourable circumstances, he can crystallize his verbal thinking beyond audible speech so that others are included in his network of communication. The tortuous invention of writing which evolved tens of thousands of years after the beginning of speech in primitive man, was epochal because it allowed ideas to be codified. Reading, or the ability to interpret those inscriptions, was also a relative latecomer in human accomplishment.

Latest of all, has arisen our awareness that some children who are exposed to formal tuition have peculiar difficulties in acquiring the art of learning to read and to write accurately and fluently.

We have tried to draw attention not to the simplicity of the topic, but rather to its complexity. When it is studied deeply, more questions arise than are answered. Our conclusions are based on the observation, examination and recording of well over 2,500 patients who were referred as putative cases of developmental dyslexia. Not all were diagnosed as such, but the majority were. Some of the children have been followed up and examined several times during a period of 12 years, and their progress assessed.

Two points became clear. One is that the syndrome of developmental dyslexia contains enough minor variations to make nearly every case a clinical collector's item. The second is that there is still very much that we do not know about the subject, and there is considerable scope for research for many years to come.

Finally, it must be said yet again that children who suffer from developmental dyslexia respond to remedial teaching of 'the right kind'. The outlook in those circumstances is far better than is sometimes supposed. Worried parents and teachers are now aware of the potentially favourable prognosis so long as the child is given appropriate help. This book does not deal with the various methods of teaching a dyslectic child to read, to write, or to spell. That is better left to educational experts, but it does set out the kind of problems to be looked for in a child with developmental dyslexia. We hope that greater recognition of the fact that such a child has difficulties beyond those of being a retarded reader and poor speller, will avoid some of the hardship which many dyslexics still experience during their schooldays.

Chapter One

Terminology

"The members of the medical fraternity can, at least, classify labelled compartments, and that, in itself, is reassuring. To be able to call a demon by its name is half-way to getting rid of him."

André Maurois

Almost every parent of a dyslectic child has at some time been made aware of overt or implied criticism of the word "dyslexia". Some teachers and educational psychologists—though few doctors, incidentally—have for one reason or another objected to that term. A few merely dislike it; some question its validity. Among the sceptics are those who assert that dyslexia does not exist; or if it does, it must be very rare and outside their experience. That the child in question is a poor reader may be admitted, but the problem is then brushed aside by saying he is a late starter who will in due course "catch-up". The mother may be regarded as being fussy and over-anxious; or it may be asserted that the child is culturally deprived at home; or that the domestic background lacks harmony and stability, and so reacts adversely upon the child; or that the family is too big. Sometimes the blame for poor reading is shifted from the parents to the child himself, who may be deemed lazy, inattentive, emotionally disturbed, or over-active. "He is not fulfilling his potential"; "Could do better", are comments which appear over and over again in the dyslectic's school-reports.

At other times, dyslexia is said to be merely the product of inefficient teaching in the junior schools, although the critics do not explain why only one or two children in the class are so affected.

Other assertions have been made, and sometimes dyslexia is snidely written off as a middle-class disorder which has become a fashionable word among parents. The headmaster of one school proclaimed that dyslexia is a euphemism for laziness.

1

Another cynic has referred to "families living at the better end of town, who run a Mercedes-Benz, whose children have braces on their teeth, one of their boys being dyslexic". This sneering remark is tragically unfair to the child suffering from developmental dyslexia.

In an attempt to explain some of the reasons for contemporary criticisms and cavilling, we will trace the history of our terminology.

For over a century, neurologists have been familiar with the phenomenon whereby brain-disease in an adult results in an impairment of his ability to speak and to comprehend the speech of others. This is the all too common condition of aphasia. The communicative powers of such a patient may not always be disturbed evenly. For example, following a stroke the ability to talk might be almost intact, but the victim may lose the power, previously normal, of understanding printed or written material although he can see it clearly, and even recognise the identity of the writer. In other words, he has lost the ability to read. "Word-blindness" was the term applied to this condition by the pioneer medical observers. Later a German nerve specialist considered that *Wortblindheit* sounded less impressive than the Greek word "dyslexia" (or alexia). All three of these expressions remained in common usage in medicine for some decades. Then in 1896 a doctor noticed that an otherwise intelligent boy suffered an isolated learning-defect which involved only the ability to learn to read, and he used the expression "*congenital* word-blindness" to describe it. Alternative terms were subsequently suggested but none attained general acceptance. An exception is "legaesthenia", meaning weak reading, a hybrid term which is currently preferred by some German writers.

Later, there was a tendency to fight shy of the word "blindness", even though it was deliberately chosen at the pioneer establishments devoted to the study and remediation of these children, namely the *Wortblindinstitutet* of Copenhagen, and the Word-Blind Centre in London (1965–1973). At least one expert spoke up for the retention of "word-blindness" as being "a good robust-sounding term, sanctioned by usage of earlier observers".

Some years after the entity of congenital word-blindness was first described, doctors and medical geneticists came to realise that some children so affected showed features indicating that the disorder was constitutional. Thus in this group there existed a clear genetic factor as well as an uneven sex-incidence. To these cases of word-blindness the adjectives "specific", or "developmental" or "specific developmental" were added.

During the 1930s, a writer whose identity is not known, suggested a less blatant expression and the word dyslexia gradually came into being, usually preceded by the adjective "congenital". This is because "dyslexia", strictly speaking, is a medical term, applied to those patients who as the result of an aphasia have lost a previously acquired ability to read.

Meanwhile, quite independently of the interest shown in this condition by medical men, who are habitually dealing with patients who suffer disturbances of function, educational psychologists began to concern themselves with the phenomenon of reading. Their researches made them aware that many children, at least ten per cent, it is said, are late in learning to read; thereafter they are conspicuously slow in making progress, and in their late teens remain poor readers if not sometimes near-illiterates. Some of the psychologists scrutinizing this group came to the conclusion that the population of backward, late, retarded or slow readers was mixed. They referred to a "continuum", within which they classified, according to their ideas as to causation, the poor readers into types. Some of the group were intellectually incapable of coping with such an artificial and tedious task as that of making sense of a series of graphic symbols. Others, it was guessed, must have something structurally wrong with the cerebrum, and, though not necessarily dullards, had perhaps sustained brain-damage at birth. However, some of the children were undoubtedly highly intelligent, and here the investigator might blame environmental factors for the child's poor scholastic progress, deeming him to be emotionally unsettled and distractable. As psychologists, their inclinations were at times orientated towards Freudian ideas, and not surprisingly some psychoanalysts came forward with their personal notions of the cause of late reading, pseudo-explanations which do not withstand the cold light of science or even commonsense.

Some writers make a distinction between "retarded' readers and "backward" readers. Thus a retarded reader has been looked upon by some authors as one whose attainments are low in relation to his age and intelligence. On the other hand a backward reader is said to be one whose reading age is less than his chronological age. One definition in Great Britain is that a reader is "backward" if his "reading quotient" is 80 or less. (Macmeeken 1939.) The matter, however, may be complicated because many children are simultaneously both backward and retarded readers, so these distinctions are unhelpful and the terms are probably best avoided.

It is preferable to speak of poor readers, slow readers, inaccurate readers, reluctant readers, seldom readers—terms which are accurate and descriptive but which do not imply any academic shortcomings.*

Educational psychologists are not medically trained. Perhaps this is why within their "continuum" of poor readers, no place was then allotted by them to the hard core of cases which doctors know occupy a special category and which constitute the real clinical syndrome of developmental dyslexia, the victims being otherwise normal, neither brain-damaged nor neurotic.

When the concept of congenital word-blindness was brought to their notice, some outside the medical profession sceptically brushed it aside as a non-existent or mythical malady. Considerable harm resulted from such a point of view, and unfortunately, the attitude of many educational authorities in the United Kingdom was adversely influenced. This view lingers on though it is steadily diminishing, for most contemporary leaders in academic and clinical psychology in this country and abroad have no doubts about the existence of the syndrome of a specialized and inborn disorder of learning, namely specific developmental dyslexia.

Mounting pressure from distressed parents, because of the large number of poor readers and by the inadequate supply of teachers to cope with all of them, led to official inquiries being

---

*The opposite state of affairs should be briefly considered, namely the notion of a "hyperlexia". This term was first used by Silberberg and Silberberg (1967), later contributions being made by Mehegan and Dreifuss (1972), Huttenlocher and Huttenlocher (1973) and Elliott and Needleman (1976). The total number of these cases has not been great.

It seems that most if not all of the children described have been been linguistically, if not intellectually, retarded, and they also show hyperactivity and various movement-disorders. Most first displayed their abilities suddenly and unexpectedly. They "read" but only in the sense of "sounding out" words, that is, without necessarily understanding them. Some of the hyperlexics read "in a compulsive, ritualistic" manner, rocking themselves to and fro. Those who have encountered such cases fail, however, to agree as to the nature and causation of the phenomenon.

instituted. Some of the reports were favourable to the concept of developmental dyslexia, others were not. At least one benefit which accrued, however, was the inclusion of "dyslexia" among the list of disorders gathered under the umbrella of "disabled persons", for whom provision was made in the 1970 Chronically Sick and Disabled Persons Act.

On the debit side, there was the Tizard Committee (1972) set up by the Department of Education and Science. It consisted of five members one of whom was co-opted; they met only four times, and nobody else was given an opportunity to present evidence. The outcome was equivocal, and the welfare of children with developmental dyslexia was in no way advanced.

The same year, the more ambitious Bullock Committee to inquire into the teaching in schools of reading and "other uses of English" was covened. Considerable evidence was taken from outside the Committee though many of those concerned with the diagnosis and treatment of children with developmental dyslexia were not invited to do so. The result was a document of 609 pages, containing as an appendix an impressive "note of dissent" of $3\frac{1}{2}$ pages. One recalls the words of an anonymous critic about another Government White Paper . . . "it reminds me of a fussy housewife who is always sweepin' and dustin', but there's never any smell of cookin' about the home". Entitled *A Language for Life* (1975), the Bullock Committee Report contains much information that may previously have been obscure with regard to the techniques of teaching. Unfortunately, upon some of the crucial issues such as the merits or demerits of i.t.a., it came to no unanimous verdict but merely temporised. When it referred to the problem of children who were behind with reading, the all-important topic of dyslexia was dealt with in eight sentences, (p. 268) which are quoted verbatim:

(1) Lastly, there is a rather smaller group of children who experience a difficulty in learning to read that cannot be accounted for by limited ability or by emotional or extraneous factors.

(2) The term "dyslexia" is commonly applied to these children.

(3) We believe that this term serves little useful purpose other than to draw attention to the fact that the problem of these children can be chronic and severe.

(4) It is not susceptible to precise operational definition; nor does it indicate any clearly defined course of treatment.

(5) Most of the children, however, do find difficulties in auditory and visual discrimination and in associating visual symbols with the sounds they represent, and it has been suggested that these difficulties are caused by delayed maturation of the coordinating processes of the nervous system.

(6) A more helpful term to describe the situation of these children is "specific reading retardation".

(7) This has been defined as "a syndrome characterized by severe reading difficulties which are not accountable in terms of the lower end of a normal distribution of reading skills".

(8) Given a skilled analysis of the nature of their difficulties, followed by intensive help and support, most of these pupils eventually learn to read, though their spelling may remain idiosyncratic thoughout their lives.*

No exception can be taken to sentences one, two, five and seven. We disagree, however, with their rejection of the term dyslexia in favour of "specific reading retardation". In fact, the Report's notion of the latter term closely corresponds with that of developmental dyslexia. The problem of the dyslexic is certainly "chronic"—if that word implies that the difficulties are long lasting. "Severe" they may be, but not necessarily so, for mild and moderate cases of developmental dyslexia also occur. It is certainly not true that the term "dyslexia" is incapable of "operational definition". Presumably, something pejorative is implied. "Operational" is a word which belongs to the disciplines of philosophy and of behaviourism. In a medical context it is out of place; "developmental dyslexia" is definable, just as much or just as little as many other entities familiar to practitioners of medicine, e.g. epilepsy, writer's cramp, headache. In other words, the argument is pedantic and untenable. Moreover, clearly defined courses of treatment undoubtedly exist and are successfully used, giving the "extensive help and support" to which the Report refers, but these features have no place in any definition.

---

* The numbering was not in the original text.

In 1968, the World Federation of Neurology promulgated a definition of developmental dyslexia. It was the product of an *ad hoc* Research Group on Developmental Dyslexia that was both international and interdisciplinary in its constitution. It reads as follows:

> "*Developmental Dyslexia*
> A disorder manifested by difficulty in learning to read despite conventional instruction, adequate intelligence, and socio-cultural opportunity. It is dependent upon fundamental cognitive disabilities which are frequently of constitutional origin."

Although not perfect, it is a good working definition.

If the "specific reading retardation" of the Bullock Committee is the same as developmental dyslexia, why is it that we regard the latter term as better? It is because "specific reading retardation" is an isolated difficulty. "Developmental dyslexia" subsumes more than a mere problem with reading; it constitutes a veritable syndrome of language-impairments. This is inherent in the etymology. "*Lexis*" is a Greek term which implies concepts beyond "reading". Its translation is "words" or, better, "the use of words". However, there has probably been a long-standing confusion with the Latin "*lexit*", which is synonymous with "he has read". If a Greek wished to specify the simple act of reading he used the term "anagnosasthenia". Dyslexia, therefore, implies not "difficulty in reading"—as so many assume—but, more precisely, all the epiphenomena that lie behind the accepted concept of developmental dyslexia. Other difficulties exist apart from the interpretation of written or printed symbols. The dyslexic cannot readily associate the sound of a word with its appearance on paper, and even when he has achieved some ability to read and to write, he often has lingering doubts as to the correct orientation of certain letters. He may experience hesitation in serial thinking, and his ability to spell usually continues to lag behind his modest skill at reading. Furthermore, a dyslexic almost always finds it anything but easy to express his thoughts fluently and rapidly on paper. Creative and imaginative, full of ideas perhaps, he is hindered when setting them down. He is also slow in copying to dictation; and at a later age he finds it difficult to take adequate notes at a lecture or meeting. Even well into adult life he may continue to be a reluctant reader, finding it simpler to absorb information by word of mouth, and also to impart it orally rather than by writing. It may well come about that his vocabulary suffers, and is not as rich as is compatible with his intelligence and degree of education, though not invariably so.

In other words, there is abundant clinical evidence to support the term "developmental dyslexia" (which represents a veritable syndrome) rather than the alternative "specific reading retardation" (which is merely an isolated symptom) suggested in the Bullock Report.

At this point it is necessary to stress that if the word "dyslexia" is used incorrectly, confusion easily arises, and because this has occurred in the past, it has unfortunately given ammunition to the non-believers. "Dyslexia"—in the sense of difficulty in coping with words—applies to more than one clinical entity. First there is the dyslexia (which is synonymous with the older term "congenital word-blindness") to which either the adjective "specific" or "developmental", or even both, should always be attached; and secondly, there is the type of reading-difficulty which is the result of structural pathology in the brain *after* the acquisition of that skill.

But, of course, there are reasons other than developmental dyslexia why some children should be late readers. A child may, for example, have been a victim of perinatal minimal brain-damage, or brain-disease in early infancy, and one of the later manifestations may well be a learning-disorder. Sometimes this is unevenly spread, so that the youngsters show among their symptoms a disproportionate problem with reading and writing, being late readers, slow readers, reluctant writers and bad spellers.

Such children, therefore, show some of the symptoms of developmental dyslexia, but the problem and causation are not the same. They belong to the category of "secondary dyslexia", which is quite a different entity. The disability is not constitutionally determined; there is no familial incidence, and boys do not necessarily outnumber girls. Children with "secondary dyslexia" may show other evidence of minimal brain-damage. They may be clumsy, poorly coordinated, inept at ball-games, beset by speech-problems, physical and mental immaturity, and a variety of other handicaps. Close physical examination by a doctor brings to light neurological signs. Most of them are indicative of brain-damage, and imperfect reading and writing are only symptoms of a structural condition. It is, therefore, a medical issue whether the physical signs found on examination represent an immaturity of the nervous system or are the expression of cerebral trauma. This will be discussed more fully in a later chapter.

It is for reasons such as these that it is always better to avoid careless references to a child being "dyslexic", without making it clear whether the case is one of developmental (i.e. primary) dyslexia, or whether it belongs to the larger group of "secondary" cases. When the distinction is clearly made, most of the objections levelled at "dyslexia" are invalid.

So far the points at issue may seem to be little more than a semantic quibble. In itself this would not be serious were it not that the unfortunate consequence of the denial of the existence of the syndrome of developmental dyslexia has been an excuse for inaction, and the victims have been caught by pedantry similar to that propounded by ecclesiastics in the middle ages who hotly contested how many angels could stand on the head of a pin. So long as discussions of this kind go on, some cases of developmental dyslexia will continue to be unidentified, and—what is worse—the victims will be deprived of the skilled remediation they so desperately need.

Chapter Two

Primary and Secondary Dyslexia: Differential Diagnosis

"If then thou wilt not read, let it alone. Some love the meat, some love to pick the bone.'

John Bunyan

In the preceding chapter, primary and secondary types of dyslexia were mentioned, and it is so important a subject that it requires to be expanded.

Twenty-three years ago, Rabinovitch isolated two main groups of poor readers, calling them cases of primary and secondary reading retardation. This seems to be the first occasion when the former expression appeared in the literature. It was not often referred to until its recent resurgence in a limited context in Great Britain. Rabinovitch used the term primary reading retardation to refer to endogenous cases of poor reading in children of normal intelligence, without brain-damage or any exogenous factors. He was probably describing what we call specific developmental dyslexia.

As defined, cases of primary, or developmental, dyslexia are of constitutional origin. That is to say, they are not the product of unpropitious environmental factors. However, should unfavourable circumstances happen to co-exist, they are likely to exercise a deleterious influence upon the child's learning-processes even though they cannot be regarded as the fundamental cause of the educational problem. Specific developmental dyslexia is inherent, innate, and genetically determined. Typically it has a familial incidence. In the case of adopted children, this is usually not known, and the grounds for the diagnosis of developmental dyslexia are less firm. When a case of developmental dyslexia occurs it would be surprising if at least one of the brothers or sisters did not have similar problems, even though it may be in an attenuated form, that is, a "dyslexia-variant" (*see* Chapter 9). The precise mode of transmission has not been established from a genetic standpoint. There was a careful study by the Swedish geneticist Hallgren (1950), and later one by Brenda Staden (1970), which is probably the most informative to date. She stated that there is a higher correlation of dyslectic fathers with dyslectic sons. Dyslectic mothers, she said, behave differently with regard to the transmission of dyslexia to their offspring. She wondered whether dyslexia is largely recessive in females but dominant in some males, and was of the opinion that mating is not a random occurrence but that dyslectic males showed a significant tendency to marry dyslectic females.

More study is obviously needed. The pedigrees of dyslectic children should be analysed to determine whether maternal or paternal transmission more commonly occurs. The factor of birth-order might also be significant, and statistics are needed to show whether or not dyslexia is more commonly found in the one-child family, or in the second born or in the last born. Although easy to ask, such questions are far more difficult for a geneticist to answer than might appear at first glance, for there are many unexpected statistical pitfalls.

In looking at family-trees it would be unusual if a case could not be found in an earlier generation, although undiagnosed but with symptoms suspiciously like those of developmental dyslexia. The affected gene may often be traced laterally as well as backwards, but it must be borne in mind that developmental dyslexia or word-blindness was rarely diagnosed more than 50 years ago and almost never in the nineteenth century. The most that a parent of a known dyslexic can sometimes assert is that a forebear "did not receive much schooling", or was "never a brilliant scholar", or that wartime circumstances militated against his education, as accounting for poor reading and spelling. Sometimes, indeed, these problems have been concealed by the family.

It is often possible to show an astonishing profusion of learning-disabilities. The following pedigrees are an illustration, some of the dyslexics therein being included in our series:

Another factor which suggests a constitutional basis for developmental dyslexia, is a characteristically unequal sex-incidence.

Boys are more often affected than girls, estimations of the proportion varying from one author to another. Some have asserted that for every girl with dyslexia there are ten boys. This

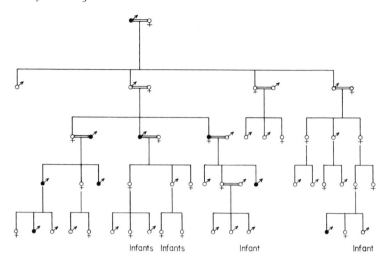

Infants Infants   Infant   Infant

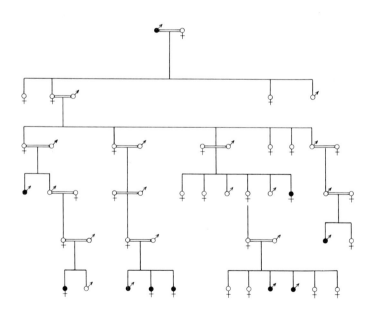

$\left.\begin{array}{l}\bullet \nearrow \\ \bullet \\ \bullet \, \text{♀}\end{array}\right\}$ Cases of dyslexia

figure seems to be too high. Out of a series of 1945 children referred as alleged cases of developmental dyslexia, 1441 have been boys, and only 504 girls. This gives a sex-ratio of 3.08 boys to one girl. Of these, the diagnosis of developmental dyslexia was confirmed in 1367 boys and 266 girls, a sex-ratio of 5.1 to one. Some critics have tried to rationalize this preponderance of males. It has been said that in paediatric practice boys outnumber girls in quite a number of diseases where the causation is known (as it is in the case of injury or infection), and which presumably are fortuitous in their incidence. Furthermore it has been alleged that a poor learner is more likely to receive greater parental concern when he is a boy than a girl, although this is probably not true nowadays.

The World Federation of Neurology definition stressed that developmental dyslexia is a "cognitive" disorder. This means that it results from some anomaly of mentation, and is not the result of any physical or structural defect in the brain. We do not know what is the pathology of the cerebral dysfunction, but just as a plant may fail to flourish without showing any tangible blemish in the root or in the soil or in the atmosphere, so many things in human biology are still unexplained.

One is tempted to invoke the hypothesis put forward long ago by Gowers of "abiotrophy"—even though the word is now unfashionable. Gowers believed that in some circumstances, and for no obvious reason, certain nerve-cells are endowed with an inherent restricted viability or limited span of vitality, and that—again for no obvious reason—such cells may perish before the expected time. So it is possible that a developing nerve-cell may be late in blossoming to maturity. Some authors have indeed spoken of the developmental dyslexic as "a late bloomer". The words are ugly, but the idea is sound.

Over the past 20 or 30 years, much of what has been written about reading-retardation has laid undue emphasis upon the influence of unfavourable home circumstances as being responsible for a child's poor ability to read. Unfortunately, this attitude has inordinately influenced the thinking of educational authorities away from any concept of inherent constitutional factors. It was implicit in the Isle of Wight Survey (1968) and in the Tizard and the Bullock Reports of 1972 and 1975 respectively.

The worried parent only too often is urged to his dismay and against his better judgement to accept that all reading-problems are closely associated with either large families, low social rank, parental neglect of scholarship and bookishness, states of near poverty, or a mediocre level of intellectual calibre on the part of the mother or father. The evidence of heredity is dismissed by some writers as merely the product of a family background of semi-literacy. Furthermore, some socio-psychiatrically orientated researchers tend to overstress the effect that parental discord and domestic conditions including broken homes, drunkenness, physical or mental cruelty, crime and profligacy have on children's reading and writing problems. The literature contains many statistics based upon surveys which unfortunately do not represent a true cross-section of the population, the samples chosen for analysis being selected. Surveys are rarely taken from a community which includes parents from social classes 1 and 2, who live comfortably in small and close-knit families, and where there exists every care and encouragement to learn. This sociological bias on the part of so many authors has produced a prejudiced attitude by some people as to the very existence of developmental dyslexia. They tend to regard it as a diagnostic label which is a face-saver or excuse for poor achievement. Developmental dyslexia occurs in all social groups but, because good diagnostic facilities are not always available, it may not be correctly identified, especially at the lower end of the social scale.

Let it be stressed once again that specific developmental dyslexia is not a defect in learning that is environmentally engendered. No one is to blame, neither the child, the parents, the teacher, nor even the social system. It is a genetically determined lag in the maturation or ripening of certain processes in mentation, and, being a relative delay in development, the handicap will in all probability lessen with time. It is foolish to assert that developmental dyslexia is untreatable. The origin of this fallacious idea can be traced back to some educational pioneers to whom dyslexia was a questionable entity, and who considered that if it existed at all it was something that was beyond remediation. Nothing could be more false, and yet these pronouncements have been accepted by generations of students of educational psychology without cavil.

Parents of dyslectic children frequently say that they have come away from interviews about their child's educational difficulties with the impression that in some way they themselves have been to blame for his disappointing scholastic progress. This is as cruel and cynical as it is untrue, when the child has a genuine developmental dyslexia. Most parents are deeply and rightly concerned about their child when, although of good intelligence, he trails behind his peers at learning to read. They take the matter to heart and do their utmost to help, even at the risk of being told that they are over-anxious and should wait patiently for the child to "mature" or "develop".

Parents should not passively accept pronouncements of this kind without investigating the matter further. They should discuss the problem with their doctors and continue to keep in close touch with the teacher, at the risk of being considered "fussy". If they meet resistance they should batter on the doors of the educational authorities, and if necessary carry their protests further.

Although the endogenous or innate nature of developmental dyslexia is all-important, it is necessary to stress that some factors certainly may exist which prove favourable, and others that are unfavourable, when the question of rate of improvement is considered.

As in the case of the acquisition of spoken speech in the growing infant, some components in developmental dyslexia can be isolated which are propitious; others are not. The linguist Miller when discussing spoken speech, stated that were we to visualize "the most precocious child orator, we should think of a blind girl, the only daughter of wealthy parents. The child with the greatest handicap would be a hard-of-hearing boy, one of a pair of twins, born into a large family with poor parents who speak two or three languages". With a little paraphrasing, his dictum can be modified to apply to cases of developmental dyslexia. We can imagine that the child with the best prognosis will be a girl born to devoted, middle-class professional parents, living in the south of England, mother and father being of the same race, sharing the same language, and with a fixed residence. Such a child should outgrow her dyslexia comparatively soon if the diagnosis is made before the age of eight; if she is not handicapped by coincidental difficulties with hearing or eyesight; if she is of high intellectual calibre; if there is access to a fully qualified teacher who is experienced in the techniques of handling dyslexics; and finally if she is a pupil at an enlightened school where the classes are small and where the concept of dyslexia is accepted. Preferably the child should be the last born of a small sibship. Most important of all, she must be blessed with those imponderable but all-important assets of determination and ambition. If she can forego the desire to excel at modern languages or the Classics, so much the better.

Later in this book reference will be made to the "prognostic pentagon".

In summary, therefore, we can say that specific developmental dyslexia is not a product of the child's environment, but a definite entity of constitutional character. To say this, however, does not exclude the fact that many circumstances may occur which assist the dyslexic towards his goal of achievement, while others prove unfavourable. These two elements, propitious and unpropitious, must be kept in mind, but they are certainly not causal.

Turning to the secondary types of dyslexia already mentioned in Chapter 1, it is usually possible to diagnose the reason for the learning disability. These cases of symptomatic or secondary dyslexia are not "constitutional", and they are not genetically determined.

One of the commonest causes of the secondary type of dyslexia has already been referred to, namely the delay in learning resulting from minimal brain-damage. Unfortunately, in the literature, dyslexia caused by minimal brain-damage has often been confused with, if not indeed regarded as identical with, the specific developmental type. One result has been to render invalid much of the statistical work as regards prevalence, the incidence of certain epiphenomena, and so on. Many authors fail to discriminate between the two kinds of learning-problem, with the result that parents often erroneously believe that because their child is dyslexic he must of necessity have suffered brain-damage in earlier life. This mistake was made in a survey of Kent schoolchildren in 1964–65. The same error probably has unwittingly been made by some writers on the topic of developmental dyslexia who lay undue emphasis upon the occurrence of "soft" neurological signs. The "Aston Index", though otherwise useful, seems to err in this fashion. "Soft" neurological signs are discussed in a later chapter.

Another reason for confusion between cases of primary and secondary dyslexia is the fact that in some respects the clinical picture of both types resembles partly that which follows disease of the parietal lobes of the brain. Indeed, when cases of congenital word-blindness first began to be diagnosed in medical clinics 70 years ago, some physicians, like Claiborne (1906), wondered whether the explanation could possibly lie in an "agenesis" or structural non-development of this region of the cerebral cortex, an area which includes the angular and supra-marginal convolutions. As late as 1958, Hermann and Norrie raised the question as to whether developmental dyslexia is a congenital variety of Gerstmann's syndrome.* Both hypotheses seem improbable (*see* Chapter 12).

A type of secondary dyslexia occurs in children whose intellectual capacity is insufficient to master the artificial task of reading and thereafter writing. It has been stated that an I.Q. of 60 is required before a child can learn to read adequately. Children whose I.Q.'s, are less than this figure cannot be expected to do so. They are dyslexic, but not primary cases of specific developmental dyslexia.

From a diagnostic point of view, the most difficult cases are the dullards whose I.Q.s', lie between 60 and 90. Most of these children will probably have learning difficulties during their school years and will lag behind others of the same age in their ability to read, write and spell because of their relative lack of intellectual equipment. Are all these cases instances of secondary dyslexia? Probably most of them are, but there is one difficulty. Developmental dyslexia, being a genetically determined and constitutional disorder, affects children of every intellectual level. Like the rain, dyslexia falls indiscriminately upon both the just and the unjust. When developmental dyslexia is encountered in children whose I.Q. is "average", "high average", "superior", or "very superior", then their low level of achievement in reading and writing is striking. But if developmental dyslexia should occur in a child whose I.Q. is 85, diagnosis becomes difficult. He is in any event a slow learner because of his low intellectual quotient. If, however, it can be clearly shown that the problem with words is far greater than with other subjects in the curriculum

---

* Gerstmann's syndrome is the name often applied to a clinical clustering of four unexpected affections, namely, (1) loss of the ability to perform arithmetical calculations; (2) difficulty in naming or identifying the fingers; (3) right-left confusion; and (4) an inability to write. Such a collection of disabilities may be conspicuous when the left parietal lobe of the brain is the seat of disease, but the status of Gerstmann's syndrome is nowadays somewhat suspect.

a case can be made out for concluding that the child has developmental dyslexia as well as a low I.Q., especially if there is a positive family history of the former.

Chapter Three

The Anatomy of Reading

"I have sometimes dreamt that when the day of Judgement dawns and the great conquerors and lawyers and statesmen come to receive their awards— their crowns, their laurels, their names carved indelibly upon imperishable marble—the Almighty will turn to Peter and will say, not without a certain envy when He sees us coming with our arms, 'Look, these need no reward. We have nothing to give them here. They have loved reading'."

Virginia Woolf

Everyone concerned with problems of dyslexia, of necessity finds himself confronted sooner or later with the question as to the fundamental nature of reading. It is important to determine exactly what is implied by that simple word "reading". A moment's thought makes one realize that the term is anything but precise, and that it is commonly used for activities which differ widely. We are at a disadvantage in not having an un-equivocal terminology, for "reading" may represent a compli-cated cognitive act, i.e. an intellectual activity; or it may com-prise merely the manipulation of a series of signals which, though not understood, can be articulated; or, understood but not articulated. For example, a phrase in a foreign language may be read aloud without knowledge of what it means. On the other hand, one may recognize what a particular Chinese ideogram stands for, but not be able to pronounce it.

Experts in the recently evolved disciplines of psycholinguistics and semeiology often go to extremes by couching their views in a way which is difficult to follow. A jargon has grown up about reading which is obscure to outsiders. Or, everyday terms may be used but in a context which is unexpected, and so they become invested with a novel or idiosignificant value.

There is, therefore, a need to set out in non-technical language just what lies behind that simple all-purpose word "reading". Even the most recondite ideas can as a rule be expressed in words comprehensible to any literate reader, for when a text is ambiguous or obscure there is a suspicion that the underlying ideas also are not clear.

Standard dictionary definitions are straightforward though perhaps they do not delve deep enough. After all, such definitions supply only lexical equivalents. Dr. Samuel Johnson defined the verb "to read" thus: "to peruse anything written; to discover by characters or marks; to know fully". As far as it goes this is excellent, but it does not take into account the declaiming of written or printed words when we do not know the meaning of them, although to do so must be looked upon as reading of a kind. It is possible to sing an aria in Italian without fully comprehending any single sentence; a Jewish boy could read aloud from his sacred scroll although he may know little or nothing of Hebrew. Such a phenomenon is referred to by linguists as "word-decoding", but even this expression is unsatisfactory, for "decoding" implies the breaking of a cipher, and, therefore, is not appropriate.

The Oxford English Dictionary goes a little further and states that the word "reading" stands for either (1) the action of perusing written or printed matter, or (2) the action of uttering aloud the words of written or printed matter. It defines the verb "to read" as (1) to peruse, without uttering in speech; or (2) to peruse and utter in speech. These definitions are better and go deeper, for they embrace and yet distinguish silent reading from reading aloud. Nothing, however, is said or even implied about comprehension. In reading, whether silently or audibly, is or is not meaning necessarily entailed? The Bullock Report of 1975 examined the matter fully. Following the practice of some contemporary linguists, the Committee could not refrain from making diagrams or little boxes, just like the aphasiologists of a century ago. Though expressed in a strained pseudo-physiological metaphor, the Report stated that three stages in the process of reading were envisaged: (a) a response to graphic signals in terms of the words they represent; (a) + (b) that is, a response to a text in terms of the meanings the author intended; and (a) + (b) + (c) that is, a response to the author's meanings in terms of all the relevant previous experience and present judgement of the reader. In other words, the three phases comprise first a "reflex"; next a "reflex" which is meaningful; and thirdly a "reflex" which is associated with perception in the fullest sense of that term. "Reflex" is, of course, a technical term taken from the science of physiology, and outside that discipline would be better avoided.

According to Goodman (1970) "reading is a selective process involving partial use of available minimal language cues, selected from perceptual input on the basis of the reader's expectation. As this partial information is processed, tentative decisions are made to be confirmed, rejected or refined as reading progresses".

Because the word "reading" means so many different things at different times, we really need a new and more precise terminology, one that is simple, unambiguous and free from jargon.

First of all, one has to consider marks on paper which differ in shape and complexity, what Oscar Wilde referred to as "black upon white . . . black upon white". What do they signify? Are they signs, or symbols, or ideograms? Indeed are they numerals, or letters, or collections of letters? If letters, what sound does each represent? Some letter-combinations, e.g. CAT, are both meaningful and vocable. Other combinations, e.g. ZXG, are both meaningless and unpronounceable. Some clusters of letters, such as *R.S.V.P.*, *e.g.*, *viz.*, *i.e.*, *etc.*, are meaningful, and yet many people make no attempt to articulate aloud the words for which the letters stand. In fact they may have no idea why the four letters "R.S.V.P." are endowed with the meaning "please reply".

It should be said that even the simple word "meaning" is imprecise; indeed to philosophers of language it is a highly flexible and ambiguous term. A dictionary definition of a word does not supply its "meaning", but merely a verbal equivalent. Ogden and Richards (1923) wrote a stimulating monograph which they entitled "The Meaning of Meaning". They pointed out that to speak of the "meaning" of a word is so vague that it is difficult to be sure that any two individuals attach the same mental associations to any given word or phrase. Other writers have made a distinction between the "sense" of a word and its meaning. However, for our purposes, the word "meaning" will be used in its broad, conventional and commonsense connotation.

The acquisition of spoken speech by a developing child is something of a miracle, the mechanism of which is still obscure for it does not entail formal teaching. Reading and writing are relatively rarer accomplishments, and require the intervention of a measure of instruction. Without such help the result is illiteracy, as evidenced by scores of millions of under-privileged people throughout the world.

Conclusion 56 of the *Bullock Report* (1974) stated: "There is no one method, medium, approach, device or philosophy that holds the key to the process of learning to read".

The steps by which a child learns to read and to write are not obvious. Many—perhaps most—intelligent literate adults who have had no specific learning-problems, have no recollection of the processes of learning to read or write and, therefore, can give no personal account of the *modus operandi* of the attainment of these two skills. As Harper Lee wrote: "I never deliberately learned to read . . . reading was something that just came to me . . . I could not remember when the lines above my father's moving finger separated into words".

Teachers are in a different position, being what the French call *assistants*, that is, onlookers as well as helpers in the learning process, and many are able to describe the earliest stages of learning proceeding from recognition of individual letters to the interpretation of whole sentences. But teaching-methods are diverse and may differ from one school to another, as well as changing from decade to decade. At times, it is tempting to suspect that a non-dyslectic child succeeds in learning to read irrespective of the procedure employed.

If the development of articulate speech in infancy constitutes a mystery, the acquisition of reading and writing is a perceptual skill which, while falling short of that standard of incomprehensibility, nonetheless constitutes an astounding attainment.

Some educational psychologists refer to a state of "reading readiness". It might be better to speak of an innate ability to acquire a literacy-skill, the fruition of which varies from one child to another. Should this endowment be weak, the result is a relative reading-retardation. When, however, the strength of the inherent ability is "normal", the skills of reading and writing are acquired with comparative ease. It has been alleged that reading-readiness is no mere passive or dormant state existing within a child, but is something that is initiated by the parent and then handed on to the teacher at the first school to foster and encourage. This may well be so.

Most children probably begin to read and write by first learning to identify individual letters and numerals. In itself this is no mean task, for most of the 36 graphic marks are empirical;

that is to say, in themselves they are devoid of meaning. The letter "H", for example, represents merely a particular phoneme and nothing else. The matter is complicated by the fact that some units of the alphabet such as "I" and "O" are shapes which can represent either a letter or a numeral. Again, sometimes in the English language, a single graphic mark can exist in isolation and yet be endowed with meaning. Thus, the letter "I" can also serve as a pronoun representing the first person singular, while the letter "A" may be promoted to the role of the indefinite article. In some foreign languages other one-letter "words" occur, e.g. "e", "y", "o", "i", as in French, Spanish and Italian; also "z" and "w", as in Polish. It is sometimes not enough in English to identify a single letter, for some of them vary in the way they are pronounced. The letter "g" could be spoken either as a hard or a soft sound. Then again, some letters are not sounded at all; the "g" in "gnat", the "k" in "knot", and a terminal "e", for example. Certain clusters of letters vary considerably in the way they sound, the most obvious instance being "ough".

From the primary task of visually identifying the letters to the secondary one of investing them with significance, there is, therefore, quite a formidable step.

As will be mentioned in Chapter 5 some children when learning their letters are handicapped—or possibly assisted—by a tendency to correlate some of them with pictorial images which have nothing to do with language. Thus, a child may associate the letter "X" with the cross of St. Andrew; the letter "I" with a pole; the letter "U" as a magnet; and the letter "O" with a hole or a hoop.

But some languages are deliberately taught in their earliest stages by using a technique of playful concretization. In Arabic, for example, the character ﻋﺞ (or *ca*) may be depicted as a fishing-hook baited with a worm, while ﻛﺲ (*ya*) is likened to a swimming duck which has just laid two eggs. In Chinese, the ideogram 口 (*k'ou*) is compared to the aperture of a squarish opened mouth. When a finger is applied to the lips thus, 中 the word becomes *chung*, or middle.

Attention will be drawn in Chapter 4 to the multiplicity of type-founts in common use. For example, a printed letter may be set out in either lower case or upper (i.e. capitals); in block capitals or in italics. Furthermore, there are many varieties of script, where the letters be joined up or isolated. Consequently a child is compelled to learn the meaning of not merely 35 different graphic marks, but more than 100.

Skill at identifying and pronouncing numerals, letters and short combinations of letters, may be achieved relatively early by some children and relatively late by others. Some teaching methods take advantage of a child's inherent powers to cope with letters as a pattern in black and white, and he is required to recognize frequently recurring groupings of letters and to identify them as a whole; or, as a psychologist might say, as a *Gestalt*. This is the idea behind the "look-say", "Aha!", or "flash" technique of instruction in reading. It is well known that many young children are able to identify certain shapes, especially if they happen to possess concrete properties, long before they can recognize words. Thus they readily learn to discriminate between coloured pictures of different kinds of animals, or birds, or even types within a particular class, e.g. dogs. They soon grasp the meaning of traffic signals. Recognition of different makes of motorcar or aircraft usually comes early. It should be noted that all the objects perceived share the property of being concrete and representational. One can imagine a stage when a child might be able promptly to distinguish and name pictures of a Persian kitten, a Siamese, tabby, or a ginger cat, and yet be at a loss to read the word CAT.

Later, the printed word CAT becomes meaningful in itself, though the child may still not be confident about discriminating it from CATS or CATTY.

Interesting results may be obtained from "tachistoscopy", which consists in the exposure of a picture for an instant, perhaps even as short as a tenth of a second, and then testing the speed of recognition. Most children acquit themselves well and succeed in identifying almost instantaneously pictures of a lion, elephant, car, bicycle, apple and so on. The same technique can be used for the flash exposure of isolated letters. In normal conditions a child soon learns to identify single letters, which are exposed at increasingly shorter periods of time. Isolated numerals are mastered earlier than isolated letters, perhaps because they are more "concrete" and represent something tangible, e.g. units of quantity, whereas a letter on its own usually means nothing.

Tachistoscopy, can also be used with groups of three, four, five or more letters. A developing child with no inherent problem with reading, learns to recognise short combinations of letters so long as they are meaningful, but he fails to pick out nonsensical clusters of letters. This distinction also applies, not surprisingly, to adults. The word FRIDAY flashed on a screen for one-twentieth of a second might be accurately identified, whereas the same letters arranged differently as RDIAFY might need to be exposed for 50 or 100 times longer before they are hoisted in as its anagram.

Data of this kind have been used to justify the look-say technique of instruction in the very young.

There is reason to believe, however, that not every learner benefits from this type of tuition. There are some who, for one reason or other, find it difficult to cope with a task which is four-fold. First isolated letters must be identified; secondly, each one has to be correctly orientated in space; thirdly, the meaning of combinations of letters must be grasped, e.g. APPLE; and, finally, the sound of the word which they know "stands for" a particular fruit, has to be correlated with its appearance in print. The developmental dyslexic is in the category of those who are slow with tachistoscopic tests.

The problem goes even deeper with the child suffering from developmental dyslexia. At a relatively early stage in the learning process, he finds difficulty in making sense of printed words, and in distinguishing DOG from GOD, TON from NOT. But with more ease he can isolate, discriminate and enumerate shapes, some of which may be quite complicated. This is the basis of the so-called Mayurama's test, where a series of cards containing nonsense-marks, superficially similar in shape but different in orientation, are shown to the testee, who is told to match the individual cards from a duplicate set, after an interval of time. (See Fig. 1.) At one time it was believed that a dyslexic would find peculiar difficulties in performing this test, but it has not proved to be so in our series. The dyslexic seems to be troubled only with verbal symbols and not with other shapes and patterns, whether meaningful or meaningless.

At this point, the experience of P. Rozin *et al.* (1971), who taught English-speaking retarded readers to learn to identify Chinese ideograms, should be mentioned. The children did so with surprising ease. In a few hours the authors succeeded in teaching eight black Philadelphian second-graders, all of whom were handicapped by a reading-disability, to read 30 Chinese characters and their English equivalents. This finding had in fact been predicted 64 years earlier by Hinshelwood, a Glasgow ophthalmologist. The work of Rozin *et al.* was collaborated by

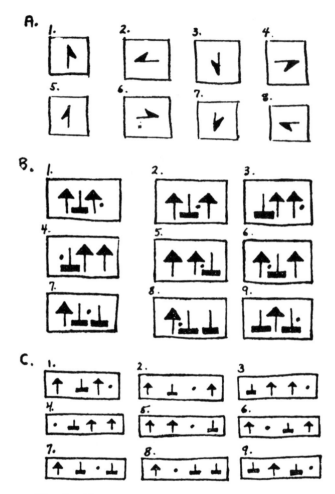

Fig. 1   Maruyama's test using non-verbal symbols.

J. E. Harrigan (1976), who tested seven first-grade backward readers in Maine. On a one-to-one basis of tuition the children quickly learned to identify from 8 to 15 Chinese characters.

As an index of progress with reading, there are numerous tests

of reading-age, some being more satisfactory than others. Some are essentially "word-recognition" tasks that explore the child's accuracy in pronouncing words when reading aloud; others seek to ascertain his skill at comprehending what he reads, whether silently or aloud; a few are claimed as doing both.

One reason why tests of the child's ability to read aloud are valuable, is that they enable the examiner to identify the nature of mistakes. In the case of a dyslexic, the errors are usually inconsistent, for he may perform accurately one moment and incorrectly the next. This nonconformity occurs over and above the handicap of the test-situation, the personality of the examiner, and the reaction of the testee.

A very noticeable feature when reading-ability is being investigated is a preliminary reluctance on the part of a dyslexic to read aloud, even when he says he enjoys reading and also that he reads for pleasure. Statements of this kind by the dyslectic child should always be accepted with reserve.

Though he may cooperate willingly in the consulting room, in the classroom his performance may be quite different as he may be reading in front of an unsympathetic supervisor as well as an audience of critical or mocking schoolmates. The whole set-up becomes highly embarrassing, and a veritable "fear of words" may develop.

As he reads aloud, the dyslectic child scarcely ever proceeds at a "normal" rate. Indeed, one of the earlier terms employed in Germany for dyslexia was "bradylexia", which highlighted the fact that the child reads slowly.

Another striking error noticeable when a dyslexic reads aloud from a printed text, is a tendency to omit words which, because of their commonplace nature, their brevity, and their simplicity, one might expect to offer little or no difficulty to him. Thus, he often skips the definite and indefinite articles. Other short words may be read incorrectly, e.g. "that" for "there"; "with" for "what". In reading aloud, the eye of any reader always runs well ahead, and the dyslexic's common fault of omitting short words may perhaps be due to the fact that in front of them he sees a longer or less familiar term which is likely to present difficulties. Anticipating a problem in identification of that long word, the dyslexic may leave out or misread the intervening short "filler", "empty", "cementing" or "utility" words. Thus, confronted with the sentence "My sister likes me to take a book and read aloud to her", the dyslectic child may say "... sister like my take book read aloud her".

During such testing procedures, the dyslectic child may lapse into his earlier tendency towards rotation of letters, and it is common to hear him say, for example, "boy" for "dog", even though he has reached the stage when the word would be spoken correctly if it had been presented in isolation. He has reversed the initial letter and guessed the rest of the word.

Another common error is to attach a terminal "s" to the end of a singular word.

Faults in pronunciation are frequent, and it is necessary to distinguish carefully between mere slips of the tongue, which may be due to skipping or skimming the text, and those errors which bear little or no relationship to the sound of the word in question. Thus when the dyslectic child in reading aloud says "particular" (peculiar), "socialist" (soloist), "officer" (official), it is probably erroneous guesswork on his part. But when he says "com-bed" instead of "combed", "wind" for "wine", "scratching" for "stretching", and "company" for "coupon", the errors are of a different nature. One suspects that in the latter case the meaning, too, has eluded the reader.

Another feature which can very often be noted when a dyslexic reads aloud is the inordinately long pauses which occur beyond the general bradylexia, indicating a mental struggle in the building up of the word phonetically. Such pauses, indeed, may sometimes be evidence that the child is, or has been, in receipt of special remedial instruction in reading, and that he is silently carrying out the procedures which he has been taught. It would, therefore, be wrong for the examiner to be overcritical in this context, without fully acquainting himself beforehand as to the type of instruction the reader has had.

There is another type of error which is of particular interest and which at first sight is difficult to explain. This is the phenomenon which may well be called "narremic substitution". That is to say, the dyslectic child is brought to a halt by a fairly long and unfamiliar word and instead of making the expected mispronunciation, promptly offers a substitution which may be a synonym or a near-equivalent. The dyslectic child may say "alive" for "healthy", "great" for "good", "beer" for "ale", "untangle" or "undo" for "untie", "anyone" for "everyone", "buy" for "bought". It seems as though he has read the word silently and has interpreted it correctly, but, for some obscure reason, supplies an audible alternative. The defect obviously lies at a superficial stage of the "preverbitum", that is, the mental operation immediately preceding articulate speech, and constitutes an unexpected fault in verbalizing a correct act of recognition. The error illustrates what grammarians speak of as "prolepsis", or the incorrect anticipation of a word resulting from an overactive "frame of expectation" on the part of the reader. Such a fault has been referred to only very rarely in the literature and then not apparently in the context of developmental dyslexia. In adults who are aphasic following a lesion of the brain, this phenomenon has been called "deep dyslexia", but the term is not appropriate in the case of developmental dyslexia.

As might be expected, the dyslexic who is reading aloud makes far more mistakes when under stress, and also when he tries to speed up his natural rate of reading.

Although almost invariably dyslexics and even some ex-dyslexics are reluctant to read aloud, especially before an audience they fear may be critical, there are a few exceptions who show the opposite phenomenon. They actually take pleasure in reading aloud a text, finding thereby that their accuracy becomes greater than when they silently and more rapidly skim the page. It seems as though audible reading acts as a quasi-controlling mechanism, or, to use the current jargon, serves as a "feedback" that exercises a favourable influence. Many older children with developmental dyslexia, especially girls, thoroughly enjoy drama lessons, or declaiming verse. They are, of course, uttering a passage which has been committed to memory, rather than reading.

When a dyslexic reads aloud, especially if he is over the age of about nine, his diction may become marred by the intrusion of a regional "accent" which is not present in his conversational speech. This may be looked upon as additional evidence of stress. The same explanation, however, scarcely applies to another feature which is sometimes encountered, namely an excessive prosody or sing-song type of elocution. A few teachers insist that their pupils declaim prose as well as verse in a manner which they look upon as being "full of expression". Nothing of the sort appears in ordinary conversation, but when this mannerism occurs in reading aloud, it still further hinders the overall performance.

Some dyslectic children—like others too, for that matter—tend to make lip-movements while silently reading. As will be described in a later chapter, it is still commoner and more obvious when the dyslectic child attempts to write.

One unusual type of reading-difficulty in a dyslectic boy of very superior intellectual calibre (I.Q. 147), who was 12.07 years of age, has been personally observed. When confronted by a page of print, he would find that his attention became riveted by the white spaces between the print rather than by the words themselves. The patterns formed in this way intrigued him. It may be that this phenomenon is not rare, but that it needs an introspective and highly intelligent youngster to bring it to the notice of others. Obviously this boy was a high-level eidetic, and he said he had had other visual experiences, such as hallucinations when dropping off to sleep, and a tendency to discern faces, forms and figures in folds of curtains and in the marks on walls, ceilings, and so on. However, no known association exists between such exquisite eidetic imagery and difficulty in learning to read, and in this particular boy the symptom was probably a coincidental epiphenomenon.

Earlier, reference was made to the fact that there are many tests of reading-age, or indices of reading-prowess, some of which concentrate on comprehension and others on correctness of articulation. The multiplicity of such testing procedures leads one to suspect that not all of them have been standardized. Indeed, workers in the field of developmental dyslexia are confounded by too many reading tests rather than too few. Some of them, and incidentally those of spelling too, were devised decades ago, and there may well be a case for checking anew their validity and perhaps discarding some of those currently in use which serve more as eponymous emblems than accurate attempts to quantify reading-ability. It must always be borne in mind that the educational pattern differs in Great Britain from that in the United States; a test used in one English-speaking country does not necessarily apply to another. Likewise, in any given language, word-frequencies are apt to change with the passage of time.

There seems to be only one reading test in the French language (known as *l'Alouette*), and one in Czech. Both comprise a series of paragraphs which have to be read aloud, and the total number of errors made by the testee is recorded. Such procedures appear over-simple. An even greater difficulty arises when one tries to collate the results from testing an English-speaking dyslexic with one from France and another from Czechoslovakia. The reading-ages are unlikely to be comparable. Reading-tests in the English language have the scientific advantage of being based upon standardized tables like the Lorge-Thorndike list, which gives a statistical index of the relative frequency of occurence of each word employed. An index of this sort does not seem to exist other than in English, so that a word-for-word translation of a foreign text would not necessarily be valid. Thus a reading-age in Czech may not represent a comparable reading-age in English. If one pursues this into the field of tests for spelling age, one finds that the discrepancy becomes even greater. How can one scientifically equate a spelling-age measured in the illogically spelt English language, with a spelling-age tested in Italian with its fixed rules of pronunciation and its richness in vowel-sounds? Even more difficult would it be to compare spelling-ages in English or in Italian with the results obtained in Polish, which has a relative plethora of consonants. More difficult still would be Hawaiian, the language being made up of five vowels and only eleven consonants.

These difficulties in correlating tests of reading and spelling-ages on a world-wide scale, make it extremely hard to assess the epidemiology of specific developmental dyslexia. Is it really so much rarer in Italy than in Great Britain, as has been claimed? Or is the rate of accurate diagnosis different? Are we, in the U.K. and the U.S.A., perhaps more alerted to its existence? Another fact which has to be borne in mind is that an Italian dyslexic may find the orderliness of his language less of an obstacle and easier to master than if his mother-tongue had been English with its erratic spelling and pronunciation. An English-speaking dyslexic, therefore, is probably a more severe and inveterate poor speller than a dyslectic Italian.

One might reasonably ask whether reading-difficulties ever occur in children whose mother-tongue is fundamentally quite unlike the structure of any European language. Chinese immediately comes to mind, because the language is not only devoid of grammar but it is not built up on any alphabetical or even syllabic basis. Like the written script of Aztec peoples and those of ancient Egypt, written Chinese consists of ideograms, some being simple, others very complex. Furthermore, unless one is conversant with etymology, there seems to exist no obvious bond linking the visual appearance of a symbol, its pronunciation, and its meaning. Each character in Chinese is made up of strokes, ranging from one to groupings of 24 or even more. A humdrum and wholly concrete idea, e.g. a horse, may be represented graphically by an elaborate arrangement of many brush-strokes, each committed to paper by a highly precise act of calligraphy. The word "nose" is *Pe*, but it is made up of 14 strokes; *Săng* meaning "to wake up" requires no fewer than 24 separate brush-strokes. Conversely, a symbol made up of two or three strokes may be endowed with an abstract and complex connotation. In either case sound plays only a subordinate role, for the auditory properties, i.e. the pronunciation of each symbol, may vary widely from one part of China to another, the "meaning", however, being fixed. It follows that a Chinese who is learning to read is confronted with a task which differs considerably from that experienced by a European child. He is faced with the problem of memorising at least 3,000 different characters. In the case of a scholar or philosopher, the needful minimum is vastly greater. The Chinese child, therefore, does not achieve reading-skill by employing any systematic process of building-up, such as obtains in English-speaking children. One might well imagine that some Chinese would find this task so difficult as to be impossible. Of course, the failure might be due to a mere defect of visual retention coupled with ready recall. On the other hand, the difficulty with reading might, from a cognitive standpoint, be entirely comparable with the problem of the developmental dyslexic of the Western world.

From personal discussion with some Chinese who are conversant with the problems of dyslexia, it seems that reading-difficulties occur in those whose mother-tongue is Chinese. Whether they are fundamentally the same as those in developmental dyslexia, is uncertain. The literature from mainland China is singularly silent on this matter.

Among the very few references available, is one by C. L. Kline and N. Lee (1976). Working in Vancouver, where there is a considerable Chinese population, they studied the incidence of dyslexia in Chinese bilinguals, brought up to speak, read, and write both English and Chinese. Their findings are in many ways surprising. This interesting paper tells us much, but not really enough, for the reader is left in a state of some confusion. The authors had the opportunity of studying 277 Chinese children attending Canadian schools. Most, though not all, came from homes where Chinese was the usual medium of communication. All of the children were learning both English and Chinese. It was found that 19 per cent had difficulties in learning to read Chinese, as opposed to 16 per cent who had difficulties of a dyslectic sort with English. Only 6 per cent had reading-problems with both languages. This low figure is hard to understand. Another unexpected finding was that reading-difficulties, in either language, decreased quickly as the children grew older. Such a rapid and marked decrement is quite unlike what one finds in English schools, and hence raises doubts as to whether all the children in the study would have been labelled in Great Britain as developmental dyslexics.

Another point arises as to the method of learning to read Chinese, and conversely of the techniques employed for testing reading-ability. To a Chinese child who is learning to read, the ideogram with which he is confronted, constitutes a pattern which he must memorize by a multi-sensorial technique. Such a task is not very different from that of memorizing shapes, and, therefore, may not necessarily impose the same type of cognitive exercise as the learning of English words. We know that dyslectic children can often unexpectedly master nonsense marks whether they are made up of Greek lettering (Fildes); Mayaruma's patterns (M. Critchley), or even isolated Chinese characters (Rozin *et al*; Harrigan). As soon as meaning is entailed, so that the signs have to be converted into symbols, difficulties arise.

A second point for consideration is the technique for testing for dyslexia in Chinese readers. Kline and Lee devised and utilized a "Chinese Iota test", the validity of which is again debatable. Apparently the child would be shown three cards to read. Card 1. contained fifteen ideograms, Card 2. twenty, and Card 3. fifteen. Superficially, these 50 characters do not seem to show progressive elaboration, nor do their English "meanings" increase steadily in degrees of abstraction.

Their intriguing paper still leaves unanswered some important questions. Does specific developmental dyslexia exist among those whose mother-language is Chinese and who are not bilingual? If so, is its incidence higher, lower, or the same as in English-speaking countries? Lastly, do there exist any scientifically quantified "tests" for poor reading and inaccurate spelling in the Chinese language?

In the context of the world-prevalence of developmental

dyslexia, one comes up against assertions that difficulties in learning to read are far rarer in Japan than in English-speaking countries (Kuromaru and Okada; Makita). The immediate reaction is that perhaps the medical and teaching professions in Japan are not yet fully alerted to the existence of developmental dyslexia. Neurologists recall that at one time it was claimed that certain medical disorders familiar in the Occident were thought to be very rare in Japan. Subsequent studies have proved these ideas to be wrong. Perhaps this holds true in the case of reading-problems.

On the other hand one must not too critically prejudge the Japanese diagnosticians. Perhaps, after all, developmental dyslexia is relatively uncommon in that part of the world. There is no epidemiological reason why such a constitutional, genetically determined disorder should not be spread unevenly throughout the world.

The nature of the Japanese written language is, of course, unusual, perhaps even unique. It is made up partly of syllabic signs (*Kana*) and partly of Chinese-style ideographs (*Kanji*). To learn to read Japanese, therefore, a child must employ a two-fold system, thus differing from what obtains in Europe and North America. Those who have had the opportunity of studying the pattern of speech-disintegration in adult Japanese aphasiacs, have found that the *Kanji* script is less vulnerable than the *Kana*. Is it, however, justifiable to use the peculiar properties of the Japanese language as an explanation of the alleged rarity of developmental dyslexia in that country?

Next we come to silent reading, which implies reading with understanding. Some tests purport to measure the degree of comprehension of a reader who is confronted with a particular text. Neale's test is often used. The reader must select the appropriate word to fill a gap in an incomplete phrase or sentence from a short list of possible terms (only one of which is applicable). This is a simplified version of a familiar test which affords a multiple choice. The child whose reading-comprehension is being tested may be shown, say, "Put the . . . and forks upon the table" and also a card upon which is a short list e.g. chairs, vegetables, knives, boots, dogs. He scores if he picks out "knives".

A test like this skims over the intricacies of perception and understanding. A moment's thought will confirm what every student of language knows well, namely that words are, at their best, imperfect tools for communication. Every substantive, however commonplace or seemingly straightforward, never means quite the same to any two persons. Thus, hearing or reading the word "table" conjures up a very personal image of a table which is not shared by others. When it comes to words which are abstract, the scope for diversity is wider. For example, the word "power" may evoke in a physicist a measurement of energy; but something very different in a politician; and in a philosopher or a poet an image that is far more allusive.

In other words, Neale's test is a rather naive and makeshift attempt to gauge the candidate's ability to comprehend.

Various levels of knowledge are required before a schoolboy or schoolgirl is able to tackle the numerous hurdles at certain stages of scholarship—11-plus, Common Entrance, C.S.E., "O" and "A" levels, degrees and diplomas. These obstacles take the place of grade-markings, internal school assessments, and oral examinations. In the case of the dyslectic student who happens to be knowledgeable, bright and ambitious, written examinations stand like sentinels, debarring him from the prizes which are his due. Such tests require that the student should rapidly and accurately comprehend the questions, and then express his knowledge on paper with fluency and speed.

Most dyslexics reach a stage when they begin to read for pleasure. They may do so slowly, but they may or may not admit it. Asked whether they ever skip or gloss over unfamiliar terms, their replies may be equivocal. The dyslectic reader probably overestimates his own reading-ability.

As stated in "The Dyslexic Child" (M. Critchley 1970), the content and the phraseology of a text raise barriers which may be too high for even a non-dyslexic to surmount. In other words, provided the reading matter is sufficiently obscure, all of us may find ourselves temporarily dyslexic. This point needs to be re-emphasized for it does not appear to be referred to elsewhere in the literature on Reading. The following passage, for example, should be within the competency of the average educated adult both to read aloud accurately and to comprehend fully:

> *"Church and State united in solemn thanksgiving. The whole land made holiday. Triple avenues of captured cannon lined the Mall. Every street was thronged with jubilant men and women. All classes were mingled in universal rejoicing. Feasting, music and illuminations turned the shrouded night of war into a blazing day."*

Turning to another text, it would not be unfair to assert that many well-educated non-dyslectic adults would be bewildered by the following:

> "*The criterion adopted for regarding a vocalization by the child as an utterance (i.e. as language) was an observable and constant relation between content and expression, so that, for each content-expression pair, the expression was observed in at least three unambiguous instances and the content was interpretable in functional terms.*"

Or, if the foregoing be deemed too technical, what of:

> "*Separate departments in the same premises are treated as separate premises for this purpose where separate branches of work which are commonly carried on as separate businesses in separate premises are carried on in separate departments in the same premises.*"

Where should this fourth specimen of prose be relegated?

> "*God's air the Allfather's air, scintillant circumambient censile air. Breathe it deep into thee. By Heaven, Theodore Purefoy, thou hast done a doughty deed and no botch! Thou art, I vow, the remarkablest progenitor barring none in the chattering, allincluding most farraginous chronicle. Astounding! In her lay a Godframed Godgiven preformed possibility which thou hast with they modicum of man's work . . .*"

At which point does the non-dyslexic find himself in the same predicament as a dyslexic in extracting meaning from what he is reading? The second and third specimens can, of course, be "excused" as fragments of professional jargon comprehended maybe by a few initiates who dwell within the communicative network. Specimen 4 is different. Most of the words are lexicon words; a few are frank neologisms or concocted words. Syntax and punctuation are strained. The quotation represents a piece of "newspeak", which was a pre-war art form acclaimed because it represented a free association of ideas.

Fortunately many genuine dyslexics are intelligent, simple and uncomplicated youngsters. The following is taken from a letter written by a dyslectic girl of 15.09 years:

> "*I find that I do not understand the questions at the first time of reading. I find that I have to re-read it and this also happens in the objective test passages. I cannot read very fast and this makes me feel that I'm wasting time.*"

The comprehensibility of a piece of prose can, as a matter of fact, be scientifically assessed and expressed as an "index of readability", to which may be added an "index of human interest". It is not necessary to quote details of how these tests are carried out: suffice it to say that a formula indicating "ease of reading" varies from 0 to 100. A high score indicates that the text is simple. Zero, or minus scores indicate that it is practically meaningless. The predictive technique takes into account such factors as word-length and sentence-length. "Human interest" scores depend upon how often there appear personal words and personal sentences. According to the linguist Miller, sentences of over 30 words need shortening before an average adult reader can make much sense of them.

In other words, written or printed material (including questions and instructions) can be made more intelligible (1) by educating the reader, and (2) by simplifying the writing. As far as dyslexics are concerned the former process must be ensured, and the latter welcomed.

Chapter Four

Putting Pen to Paper

"The first day home from school, little Milton's mother ran out eagerly to meet him. 'So what did you learn?'. 'I learned to write,' said Milton. 'On the first day already you learned to write? America gonif! So what did you write?'. 'How should I know?' said Milton. 'I can't read'."

Leo Roster

Penmanship.

A dyslexic's difficulties in reading are reflected, as in a lake, by defects in his written work. Ajuriaguerra and Auzias (1975) well said that writing difficulties are no more than the magnifying glass of various problems; that is certainly true of a developmental dyslexic. Both his reading and writing are cluttered with errors, some of which can be analysed and measured. In the case of the teenage dyslexic, the faults in writing greatly exceed those perpetrated in reading. The number of mistakes is far greater than one would associate with the intelligence and the chronological age, and corresponds more closely with the reading age, though nearly always lagging behind.

An experienced examiner can often glance at a sheet of spontaneous writing and make a shrewd guess that the writer is, or has been, dyslexic. This judgement is not based upon the finding of any isolated factor which can be deemed specific or pathognomic, but stems from a combination of those shortcomings which give an overall picture recognisable as the work of a dyslexic. A handwriting expert calls this the "form level" of a page of script.

In the first place, a dyslexic—even an "ex-dyslexic"—is rarely a rapid writer. Slow writing, or what the Germans call "bradygraphia", characterizes the handwriting—whatever the circumstances of its performance. It applies to the slavish copying of a text placed before him; it holds true for writing to dictation, and still more so for spontaneous writing. It may bedevil his attempts to take notes at a lecture. Because of this slowness, the teenage dyslexic has difficulty in completing within a set time, adequate answers to examination questions, and often a sense of urgency adds to his distress. This anxiety is not due to lack of knowledge on the part of the candidate, but to his inability to express himself satisfactorily on paper in the allotted time. Failure to write with facility shows itself well in the stereotyped and often brief letters which the dyslexic at a boarding school sends home each week to his parents. Sometimes he does not write at all, preferring to communicate by telephone.

Slowness in copying can be measured, as described later in this chapter.

Graphologists record the speed of writing, including copying, by estimating what they call the C.P.S. or number of "characters" per second. A "character" is not the same as a letter, for while each individual letter is accorded one point, a point is also given to a space as well as to a punctuation mark. All upper case letters, an "i" which is dotted, and a "t" which is crossed, are each rated two points. The transition from the end of one line to the start of the next is also given two points. Consequently the word "character" is misleading, and would be better replaced by some such term as "graphic unit". For example, in the following phrase, "The book you want, is *Our Mutual Friend*", there are 31 letters, but the number of graphic units ("characters") is 50.

One graphologist has estimated that in the handwriting of non-dyslexic adults, the graphic unit per second (or G.U.S.) ratio lies somewhere between 2 and 5. In another series, which included school children, the mean G.U.S. was said to be 3·3.

In a dyslexic's writing, slowness can be detected because the penmanship bears the hallmarks of slow writing. Electrical methods exist for recording the rate at which a piece of writing has been executed, and such techniques have been used for detecting forged signatures which, as might be expected, have always been carried out slowly. In assessing the handwriting of a dyslexic, such elaborate measures are unnecessary, for the rate of writing is obvious to the experienced eye. A regularity or smoothness characterizes slow writing, each individual letter being complete in shape. By contrast, rapid writing is less uniform, although of course exceptions occur.

Adjacent letters show an accurate linkage. The joining-up of successive letters is technically spoken of as a "juncture". These vary from one writer to another, and graphologists classify the

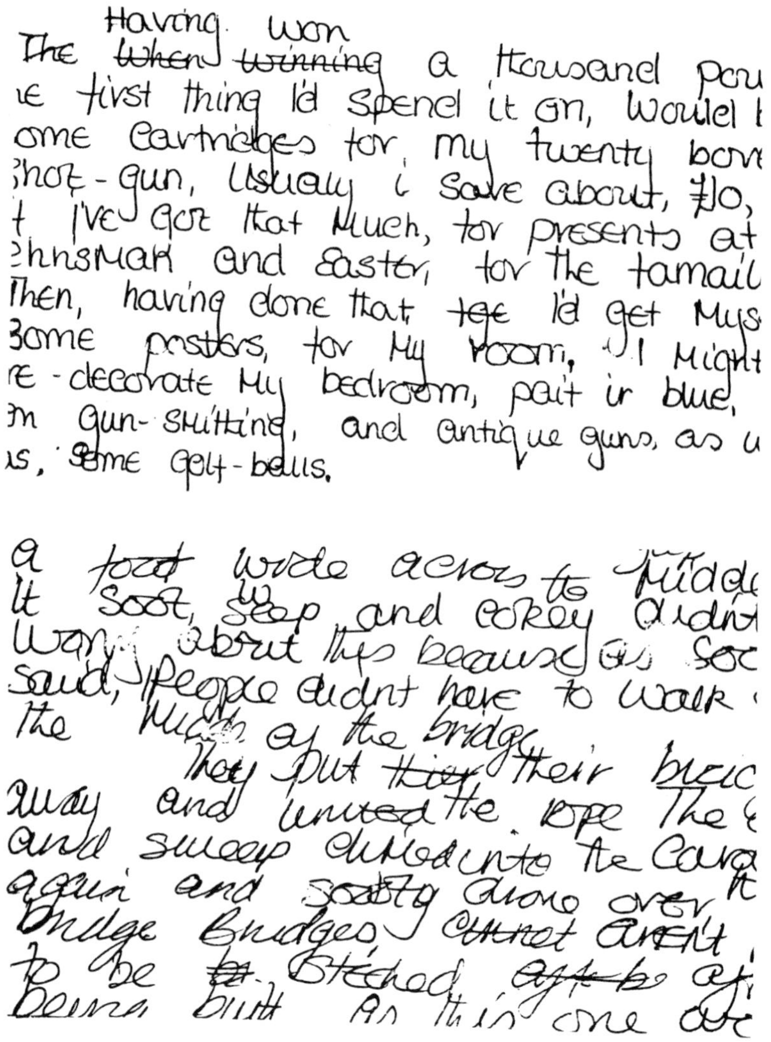

Fig. 2 Comparison between (above), slow writing of a boy, aged 15.09 years, with resolving dyslexia (taken from an essay), and (below), his rapid copying of a printed text. Speed of copying: GUS 2.62. (RA 14 +; Sp.A; − 14; Full scale IQ 98).

common patterns as "arcades", "garlands", and "angulations". It must be remembered, however, that in some Junior schools, junctures are not taught. The child might be taught to print words with the constituent letters disjoined, and not until later does he learn to write in a "joined-up" or cursive fashion.

The amount of pressure of the pen on the paper varies inversely with the speed of writing. Heavy pressure is usual in slow writing and is easily detected if an old-fashioned ink-pen has been used. In script written with a ball-point pen or a pencil, the signs of pressure are less obvious, but they can be emphasized by placing a sheet of carbon paper under the top page. When the writing is carried out slowly, the carbon copy exaggerates the differences between the heavy down-strokes and the lighter up-strokes, especially in "upper and lower zone" letters (e.g., h and y). Such features are common in the writing of dyslexics.

In both copying and spontaneous writing when pen and ink have been used, slowness is betrayed by yet another characteristic, namely frequent pauses. After a few words the writer may momentarily halt and even lift the pen off the paper. These stopping places, and the lifting of the pen show up distinctly in ink, but less so when a pencil is used.

A most important criterion of the rate of writing is the nature and employment of diacritics, that is, the dotting of the letter "i" and the crossing of the "t". Thus, the slow writer usually places the dot accurately and not too high above the "i", whereas the rapid writer, if he dots his "i's" at all, does so as an after-thought. His belated jerking movement may be wide of the letter "i", or he may substitute the dot by a short oblique bar or stroke. However, many a young dyslexic consistently fails to dot his "i's" and less often to cross his "t's", not because he is a fast writer but because he is dyslexic. Although writing slowly, he displays some of the sloppiness of the fast non-dyslexic.

The manner of crossing a "t", or of forming this letter as a whole may be an eloquent witness of hurry. The rapid writer distorts the letter in various ways. He may extend the horizontal bar well to the right of the vertical stroke; or he may elongate it unduly. If the dyslexic uses the (*t*) form he may deform it almost out of recognition, even though it has been written slowly.

Another feature which betrays both slowness and immaturity of writing is an inordinate gap between successive words. Spaces separating one word from another may be as wide as fifteen or even twenty millimetres, and we often observe this in both the spontaneous writings and the copying of dyslectic children.

Most young children, and certainly the majority of dyslexics, write in a large hand. As a rule, they outgrow this practice, but

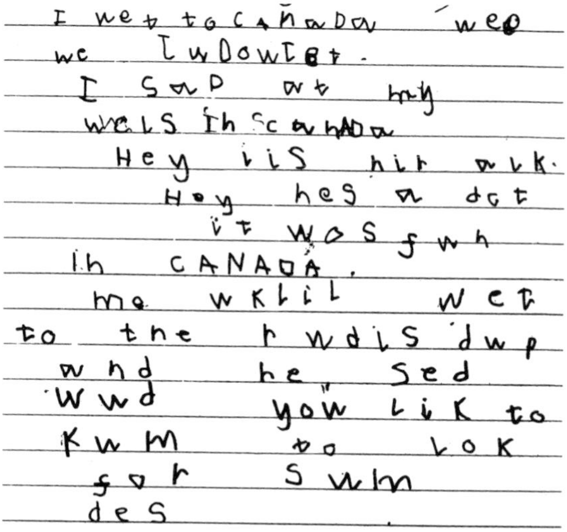

I went to Canada we went in a jumbo jet
I stayed at my uncles in Canada
They have a boat   It was fun in Canada
My uncle went to the rubbish dump and he said
would you like to come to look for some bears

Fig. 3 Essay written by a dyslectic boy of 7.09 years. (R.A. — 6; Sp.A. 6.06).

dyslexics are slower to do so. According to graphologists, writing can be considered as "large" when the height of the middle zone letters ("a", "c", "e", "i", "m", "n", "o", "r", "u", "v", "w") is 4 mm or more.

Other personal idiosyncracies are to be seen in the penmanship of both dyslexics and non-dyslexics. The degree of "slope" in the writing of a young child is influenced to some extent by the manner of holding the pencil, and also by the way he has been taught. "Upright writing" subtends an angle 75°–95°; less than 45° is regarded as "very sloping", and over 95° (i.e. tilted to the left) is spoken of as "recursive". National standards of penmanship play a role. In the U.K. an angle of 70°–90° is conventional; in the U.S.A., 60°; while in France, handwriting commonly slopes still more to the right, with a writing angle of perhaps 45°.

Writing which is strictly vertical, sloping neither to right nor to

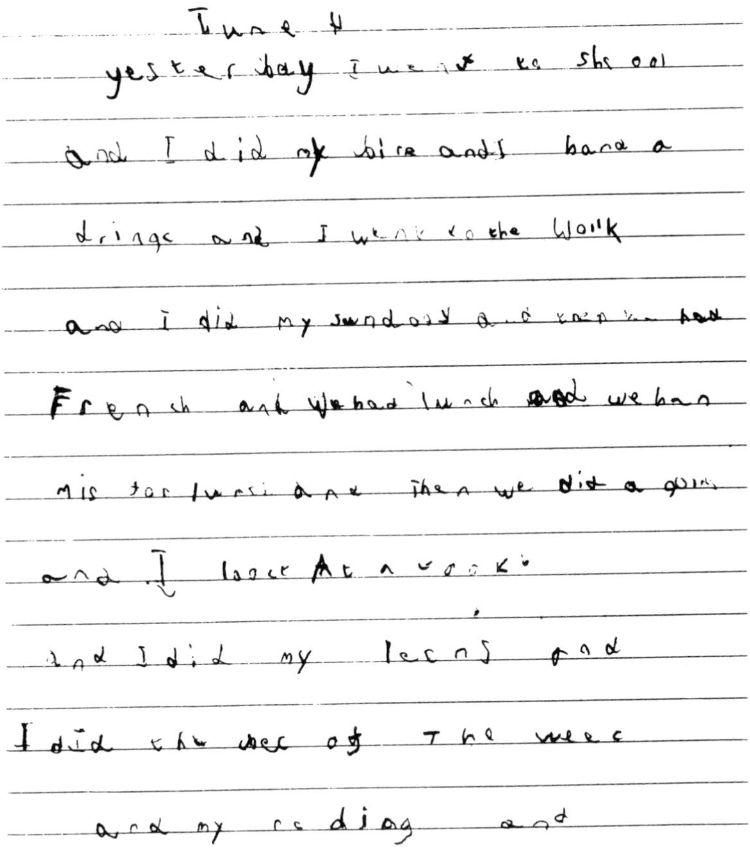

June 4
yesterday I went to school
and I did my diary and I have a
drings and I went to the Walk
and I did my sundary and then we had
French and we had lunch and we had
mis for lursi and then we did a quim
and I look At a book.
and I did my lesns and
I did the week of The week
and my reading and

JUNE 4th

Yesterday I went to school and I did my diary and I went to the walk and I did my sum book and then we did French and we had lunch and we wrote a poem and I read a book and I did my lessons and I did the days of the week and my reading and I went downstairs to Mummy took me to Paddy's house and I made a model and I went to Adam's house and then I went back home.

Fig. 4 Essay written by a dyslectic boy of 6.11 years. (R.A. — 6; Sp.A. 6.06). Note isolation of letters and wide gap between adjacent words.

left, usually implies a slow writer, and hence is fairly common in
the essays and notes of a dyslexic. Until maturity a dyslexic may
write capriciously, with some words vertical, other words sloping
a little to the right, others to the left. Inconsistency of this sort
characterized the penmanship of Balzac, who admitted, "I have
as many handwritings as there are days in the year". There is no
evidence that he was dyslexic, however. On the contrary indeed. He was an unsatisfactory pupil, but an omnivorous reader.
In his semi-autobiographical novel *Louis Lambert* he wrote that
"reading was a sort of appetite which nothing could satisfy. . . .
He devoured books of every kind, feeding indiscriminately on
religious works, history and literature, philosophy and physics.
He had told me that he found indescribable delight in reading
dictionaries for lack of other books . . . His eyes took in six or
seven lines at once."

Rather surprisingly, the effect of schooling upon the style of a
child's handwriting is less than might be expected. Skilled graphologists are able to identify personal qualities in the writing of
children even as young as six or seven years of age. Graham
Greene was aware of this fact when he wrote "even our handwriting begins young and takes on the tired arabesques of time".
According to the graphologist, H. J. Jacoby, "every child imbues
the school-model with his own expression, his individual vitality".
This personal independence in style may possibly be even more
marked in the case of a dyslexic than it is in non-dyslexics. It is
probably more conspicuous today than it was a couple of generations ago, when greater attention was paid in instructing a child to
write in a neat and acceptable style.

As he approaches adulthood a child often changes the form-level
or general pattern of his writing, so that with increasing maturity
he develops a style which is individual. This applies to dyslexics
and non-dyslexics alike. But in the former, minor variations can
be observed even in the course of a single day, the writing being
more influenced by such factors as fatigue, hurry, ill-health, or
stress. Handwriting experts emphasize, however, that such fluc-
tuations are relatively superficial, and that no writer can ever dis-
guise the fundamental characters of his writing. Identification is,
therefore, always possible. Penmanship is like a landscape which
remains basically unchanged despite passing tricks of cloud, mist,
sunshine and twilight.

When one studies the spontaneous writing of dyslectic children other anomalous features may be discerned. It is not uncommon for a dyslexic aged between about 10 and 15 years to write, albeit slowly, in a fashion which is almost undecipherable. The principal cause of the difficulty in comprehending the text lies in inaccurate spelling, a subject which will be considered later in this chapter. Some of the errors are phonetic and can be interpreted with no great trouble. Other spelling mistakes are bizarre and offer no clue as to their meaning. Not only does the reader fail to make head or tail of what has been written, but the child himself often cannot read it back, unless, of course, the subject-matter has been firmly retained in his memory.

Doubts and second thoughts by the writer as to spelling are evidenced by the numerous erasures and crossings-out, but rarely are the corrections sufficient to embrace all the errors.

Difficulty in deciphering the writing of a dyslexic also results to some extent from malformed letters. Strange fusions may connect one letter with the next so as to produce an unconventional symbol (Figs 5 and 6), even when the penmanship is otherwise acceptably neat.

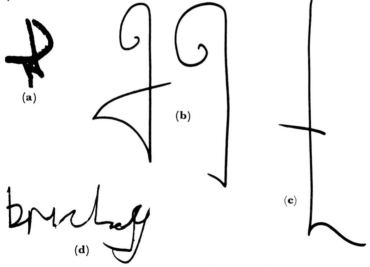

Fig. 5   Distorted letters penned by dyslexics:
(**a**)   Letter "G".   Male aged 8.09
(**b**)   Two versions of the word "of".
Female aged 17.03 (R.A. 14; Sp.A.13)
(**c**)   Letter "t" written by same girl.
(**d**)   The word "bridge". Male aged 8.02 (R.A. — 8; Sp.A. — 8)

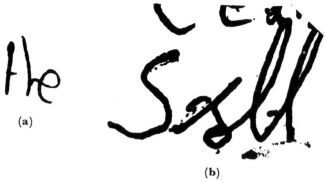

(a)

(b)

Fig. 6 (a)   Fusion of the two consecutive letters "h" and "e" in the word "the". Male aged 13 years. (b) Fusion of letters; omission of letters; neographisms, illustrated in the word "School". Male, aged 12 years.

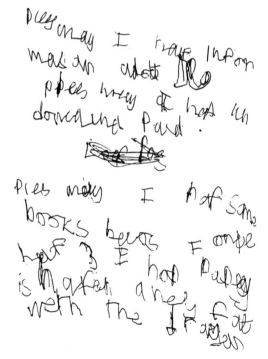

Fig. 7   Barely legible spontaneous writing by a dyslectic boy.

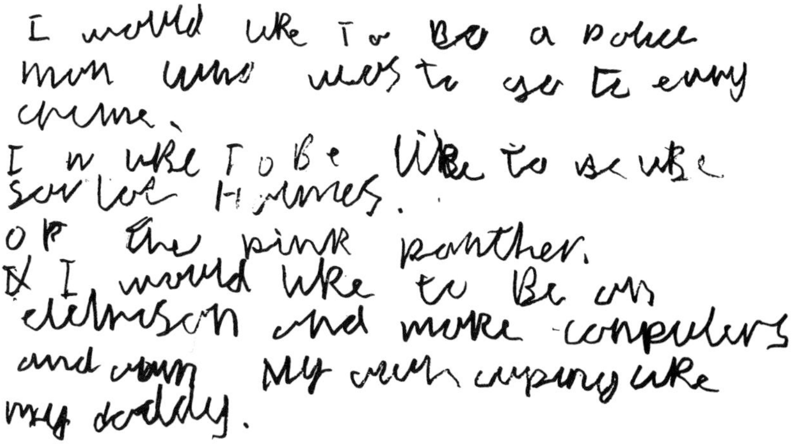

I would like To Bo a police
mun who wos to ser te evry
cheme.
I w uRe To B: lRe to scuBe
sov loe H jnnes.
oP the pink panther.
& I would uRe tu Be ons
clemson and mure -conpulers
and vum Ny own cupiny uRe
my daddy.

Fig. 8 Essay, written without supervision in the space of five minutes, by an atypical dyslectic boy aged 8.04 years. (R.A. 9.09; Sp.A. 8.03).

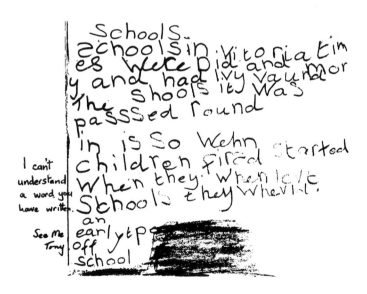

Fig. 9 Spontaneous writing by a dyslectic boy of 8.09 years. (R.A. 7.09; Sp.A. 7.09). Note the teacher's comments in margin.

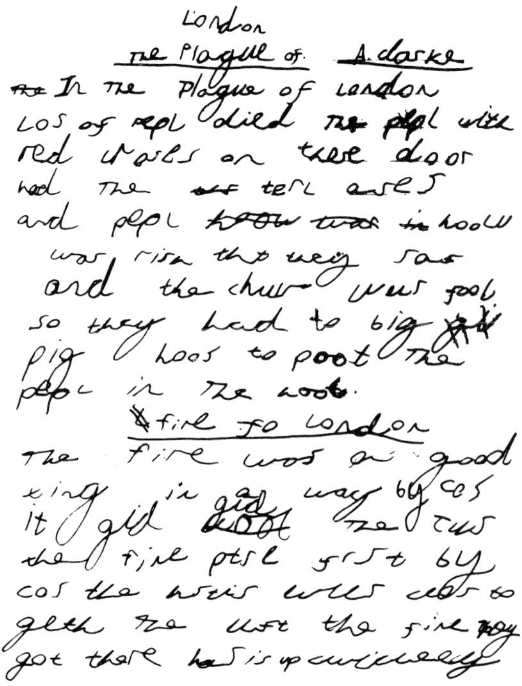

Fig. 10   Spontaneous essays by dyslectic boy
aged 10.04 years. (R.A. 6.06; Sp.A. 7 +).

Typically, the written work of a dyslexic is notable for its brevity; the relatively large size of the letters; signs of slow execution;
wide spacing between words; and tortured penmanship. To these
characteristics may often be added: deviations from the horizontal
even to the extent that two successive lines merge; deformation of
letters and clusters of letters; frequent erasures; copious mistakes
in spelling; misuse of punctuation; lack of paragraphing; and an
intrusion of upper case letters within the body of the word.

Some dyslexics are taught at a relatively early age to use a type-
writer. This is not without merit if only because it throws into
bolder relief the faults in spelling, and the dyslexic cannot so easily
conceal orthographic doubts by resorting to untidy writing. Thus,
having to spell the word "niece", he may be unsure whether or not
it should be written "neice". As a cover up, his handwriting may
deteriorate at the appropriate moment to such an extent that the

PLATES 1–3

Mysterious

The ~~Misterest~~ sun

In ~~the~~ summer one year the sun shone
very ~~weekly~~ *weakly*, and nobody could get a tan.
~~how~~ ~~have~~ ^*however they* hard ~~you~~ tried.

But, one day, ~~in~~ the Newspaper ~~said~~ said,
"A YOUNG POOR ~~COUPLE~~ *couple has* ~~HAVE~~ BEEN
SCORCHED by the sun~~one day~~."

Every ~~body~~ said "That they couldn't become
brown". Then after that a scientist looked
at the sun and said, "That is the *poorest* ~~lowest~~
~~climate~~ I have ever seen," It was so dim
thats ~~you good see it~~ *impossible*.
Every ~~body~~ said, "~~it is~~ ~~unprobable its~~ It's
not true, they have been ~~away~~ *abroad*."
They ~~replied~~ ~~repled~~ "We can not ~~offed~~ *afford* to go
away" the scientist ~~examine their~~
Then ~~the scientist came to~~ ~~examine~~ there
cottage. The sun shone ~~terbly~~ *terribly* brightly on
their ~~hous~~ cottage.

Then, after they had been inside
the cottage, they went outside. Then
they studed the + garden and as they

Plates 1 and 2 Essay written by a dyslexic of 10.02 years. R.A. 10.03,
Sp.A. 9.03. Teacher's comments and corrections are in red.

went round they ~~noted~~ noticed a small gaget on the garden wall. ~~and~~ If you were one meter away or more it would tan you. Soon the ~~police~~ came round to arest them and to take them to court. When they came in and the ~~Judge~~ started asking them questions he ~~pleed~~ pleaded ~~innosent~~ innocence. Then the ~~scietists~~ said "the technolgy is too clever for any human-being". Then the couple went home to their cottage and, as they went in there, they found a little ~~Marson~~ Martian (that's what they ~~thought~~ anyway) and it said "8 8 @ 8" then the couple looked at each other in ~~great~~ ~~asonasment~~ great astonishment. Then the ~~scietists~~ came round and said "we found ~~their~~ space - ships and mended it. We ~~ar~~ are taking them now." They took off

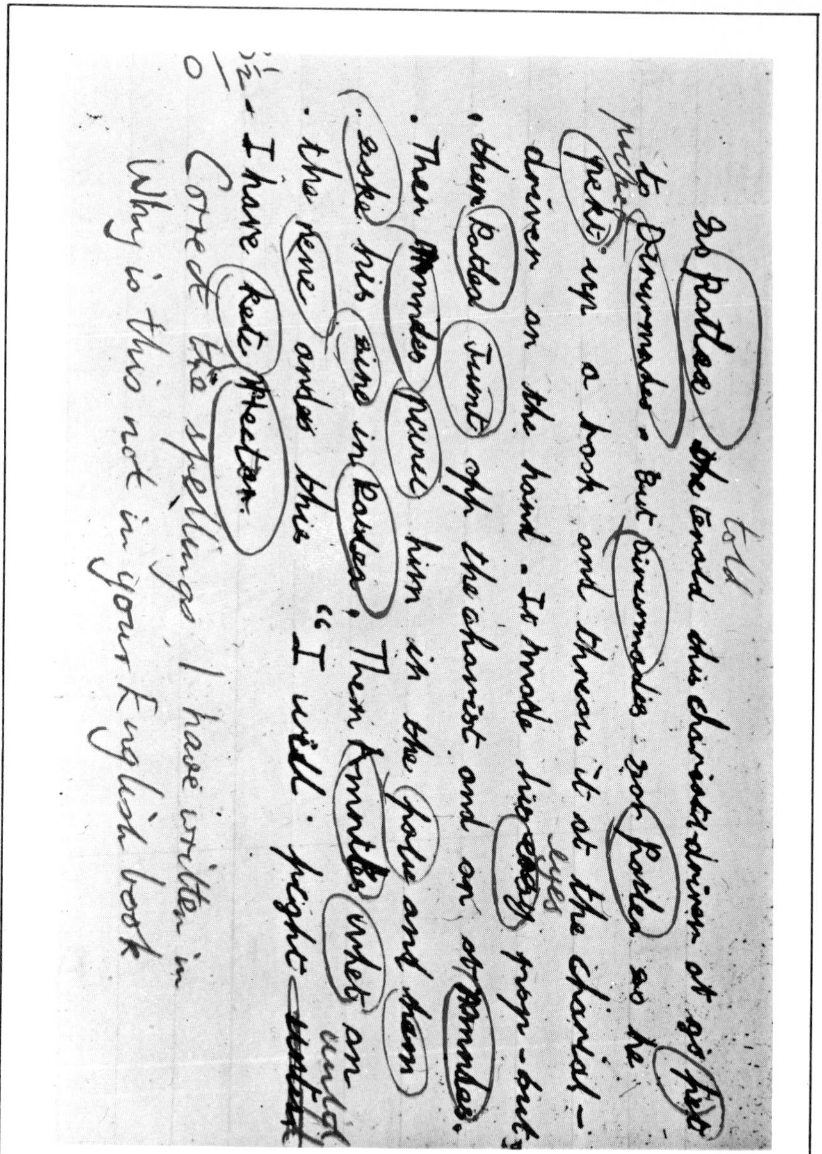

Plate 3 Letter written by a dyslexic of 11.09 years. R.A. 7.06, Sp.A. —7, Teacher's comments in red ink.

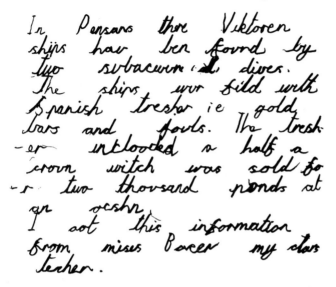

Fig. 11 Spontaneous writing by a dyslectic boy aged
10.11 years. (R.A. 9; Sp.A. 8).

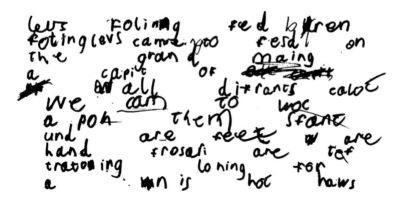

Fig. 12 Spontaneous writing of a dyslectic boy of 8.06 years.
(R.A. 7.06; Sp.A. 7).

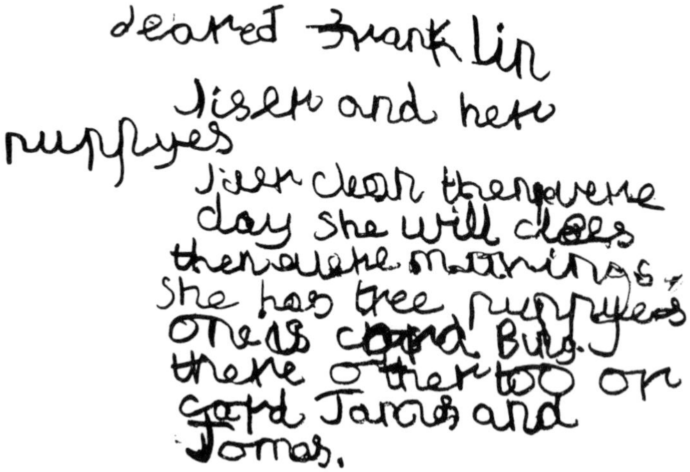

Fig. 13   Story written by a dyslectic boy of 8.08 years. (R.A. 6.09; Sp.A. 7.06).

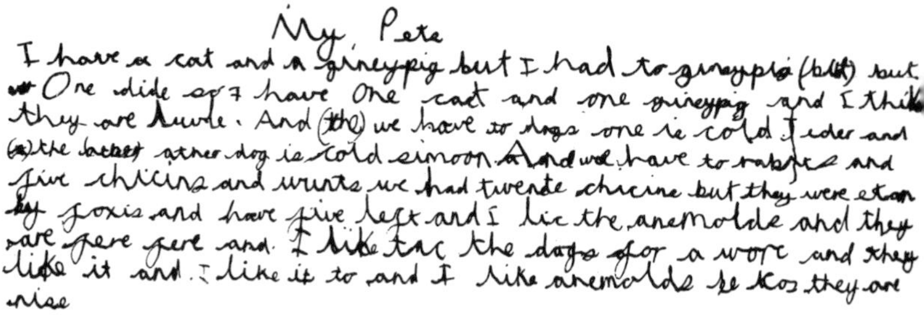

My Pets

I have a cat and a guinea pig but I had two guinea pigs but one died so I have one cat and one guinea pig and I think they are lovely. And we have two dogs one is called Jedha and the other dog is called Simon. And we have two rabbits and five chickens and once we had twenty chickens but they were eaten by foxes and have five left and I like the animals and they are very furry and I like taking the dogs for a walk and they like it too and I like animals because they are nice.

Fig. 14   Essay written by a dyslectic boy of 8.09 years. (R.A. — 6.06; Sp.A. 7).

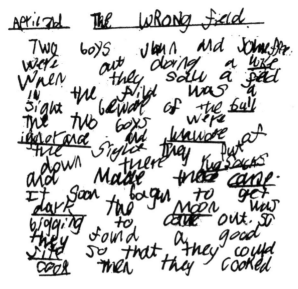

Fig. 15   Essay written by an atypical dyslectic
girl aged 9.07 years. (R.A. 13; Sp.A. 9).

reader cannot determine whether he is viewing "ei" or "ie".
When typing, a potential mistake cannot so successfully be covered
up.

Nevertheless, a page of typescript executed by a dyslexic,
whether spontaneous, to dictation, or copy-typing, is liable to be-
tray a considerable number of errors. Among the defects likely to
be found are irregularities in alignment; misspellings, only some of
which may have been detected and corrected; lack of spacing
between successive words; linear inequalities; and serious errors in
punctuation. The dyslectic typist is obviously alive to some of the
faults perpetrated as witnessed by the alterations, but obviously
many if not most of them have escaped attention. (see Fig 17)

Some adolescents show so much discrepancy between a relatively good reading age and distorted written work, that a few
writers have been tempted to invoke the notion of a "developmental dysgraphia". It is not certain, however, whether enough
data exist to warrant the idea of an isolated or specific disorder of
writing wholly independent of difficulties in reading. Until evidence to the contrary is forthcoming, it would be better to look
upon these cases as lying within the province of specific dyslexia.

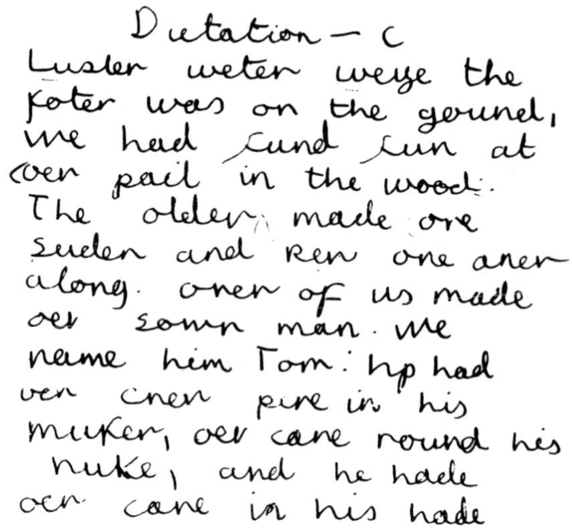

Ductation — C

*Luster weter weye the
foter was on the gorund,
we had fund fun at
oen pail in the wood.
The olelev; made ore
suelen and ken one anen
along. onen of us made
oel somn man. we
name him Tom: hp had
ven cnen pure in his
muxen, oel cane round his
nuke, and he hade
ocn cane in his hade*

Last winter while the frost was on the ground, we
had fine fun at a place in the woods. The older
children made a slide and pushed one another along.
Others of us made a snow man. We named him
Tom: he had a clay pipe in his mouth, a chain
round his neck, and he held a cane in his hand.

Fig. 16   Writing carried out to dictation by a dyslectic boy aged 9.11
years. (R.A. − 8; Sp.A. − 8).

There might originally have been a slight reading problem which
could have been overlooked at the time or even forgotten in later
life.

When embarking upon the difficult task of writing, children
may adopt awkward bodily postures. An attitude of crouching so
that the nose almost touches the page is familiar enough, but
whether this applies more so to dyslexics has not been established.
(See dust jacket illustration). To quote Charles Dickens:

> "... she soon occupied herself in preparations for giving Kit a writing lesson
> on which it seemed he had a couple every week and one regularly on that
> evening to the great mirth and enjoyment both of himself and his instructress
> ... His sitting down in the parlour in the presence of an unknown gentle-
> man—how when he did sit down, he tucked up his sleeves and squared his
> elbows and put his face close to the copy book and squinted horribly at the
> lines—how from the very first moment of having the pen in his hand, he

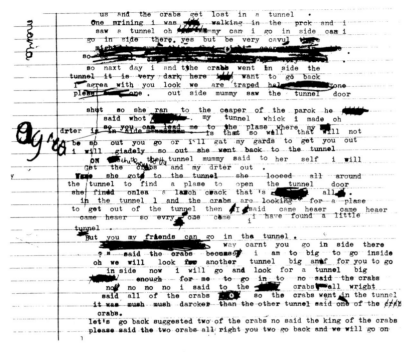

Fig. 17 Typewritten story by a dyslectic girl aged 9.02 years. (R.A. — 8.09; Sp.A. — 9).

began to wallow in blots, and to daub himself with ink up to the very roots of his hair—how if he did by accident form a letter properly, he immediately smeared it out again with his arm in his preparation to make another—how at every fresh mistake, there was a fresh burst of merriment from the child and a louder and not less hearty laugh from poor Kit himself".

It may well be that it does occur more often in dyslexics, for the phenomenon is certainly a badge of literary immaturity. In a few young dyslexics, small-range movements of the lips may be so exaggerated as to mimic a chewing, a smacking, or a munching, reminiscent of the tic-like mouthings of some old people. Do these movements in some way assist the apprentice writer as he wrestles with his uncongenial, unfamiliar and irksome task? If so, he might find himself in even greater difficulties were these movements to be artificially restrained. Darwin (1872) was probably the first to suggest that these tongue-twists assist a child in his efforts to write. Nasarova (1955) also directed attention to these motions, which she called movements of "co-articulation." If inhibited artificially, she said, the incidence of mistakes in writing might materially increase. Some of the young dyslectic patients in our series were asked to hold a pencil in their mouths, close their lips and teeth firmly upon it, and then try to write with another pencil. Were Nasarova correct, the performance should thereby be rendered still more awkward. However, no such worsening was found in any dyslexic tested in that way. Such a negative finding was a little surprising, because in adult patients with acquired dyslexia following brain-disease and showing co-articulatory lip-movements, the pencil-in-mouth test appears to be inhibiting. (Personal observation, A. R. Luria and M. Critchley, in Moscow in 1964).

Regarding the act of writing it must be realised that every left-handed individual experiences a relative impediment, unless he is expressing himself in an Arabic, Hebrew or Iranian script. Should the sinistral also happen to be dyslexic, these detriments are enhanced. The natural tendency for the writing-hand, whether right or left, is to proceed in an abductive direction, that is, outward from the midline. This is not simple even for a child who is learning easily to read and to write. It is still more difficult for the young dyslexic who is already confused as to the lateral dimension of an individual letter, and he may reverse the direction not only of isolated letters, but even whole words. The result may be mirror-writing. At times, indeed, parents and teachers are first alerted to a child's reading-difficulties by the frequency with which he produces mirror-script (which, incidentally, he can usually read with no greater and no less difficulty than orthodox writing or print).

Sinistrals often simplify the act of writing by turning the page through an angle of 90° usually to the right, less often to the left. The result is that the left-hander writes vertically, either upwards or downwards. Whether this style is commoner in sinis-trals who are also dyslexics cannot yet be asserted with confidence.

A left-hander also finds that his left hand obscures and even smudges words that have just been written. To obviate this, he may adopt an unorthodox manner of holding the pen. He may rest the forearm above the writing line and then overflex the wrist. This is the so-called "hook-posture". In this way the point of the pen is directed towards the chest instead of away from it. Whether the hook-posture is found more often in left-handers who are, or

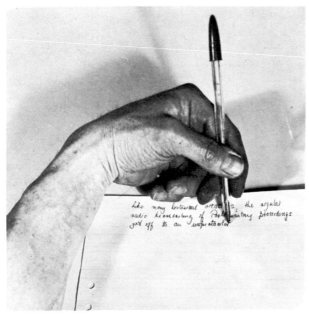

Fig. 18 The "hook posture" adopted by the wrist and forearm of a sinistral during the art of writing.

who have been, dyslexic, is not known, but it may well be so. Levy and Reid have come forward with some interesting, though speculative, ideas on the subject. They have hypothesised that there is an equipotentiality as regards the function of the two halves of the brain, surmising that those who hold their pens in this manner have speech-centres on both sides of the brain, unlike the usual state of affairs. This notion has some bearing upon Orton's ideas of the aetiology of dyslexia.

These unorthodox ways of holding the pencil or pen are apt to be reflected in the script of any left-hander. Perhaps they are merely bad writing-techniques and are irrespective of reading difficulties.

We now come to the phenomenon of "make-believe writing" which is occasionally indulged in by very young dyslexics. At a distance and at first glance such pseudo-writing looks like a genuine piece of script, for it is set out in parallel lines, with margins to right and to left; there is an irregular fragmentation in the writing giving the appearance of words, and a succession of

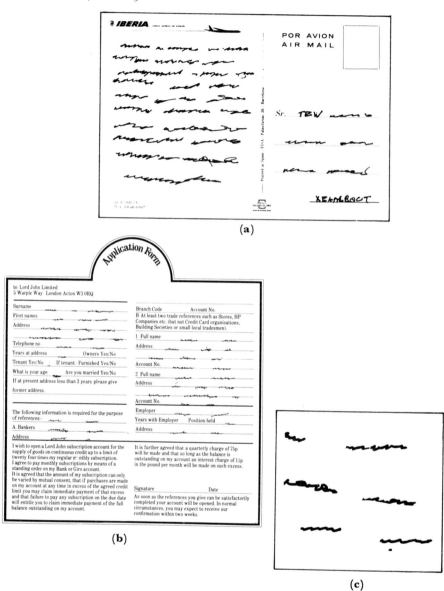

Fig. 19 (**a**), (**b**) and (**c**)   Make believe or pentecostal writing executed by a dyslectic boy aged 7.06. (R.A. 6.03; Sp.A. 7). When last seen, aged 11.05, he no longer indulged in this type of writing and had a R.A. 10.09; Sp.A. 8.06.

upper and lower zone symbols intercepting the middle zone markings. Nonetheless, the script is wholly indecipherable. The writer may even "address" an envelope in a plausible fashion with three or four successive lines, appropriately inset, and finishing with what seems at first sight to be the name of a city or county (see Fig. 19).

A child who produces this kind of script has evidently taken pride in penning the make-believe "pentecostal" writing, as it may be called, and he often shows a compulsion to inscribe many sheets of paper in this way. Such a dyslexic may even execute make-believe writing "out of sight", that is to say, in the dark or under the bedclothes. This interesting phenomenon is not common, but perhaps it may be looked upon as a favourable omen for the future, for it might be a hallmark of an innate and powerful desire to master the art of writing. Such an attitude is certainly preferable to the *non possumus* reaction of some other dyslexics who stubbornly insist that the task is beyond them.

Such a simple explanation would not, however, satisfy all psychoanalysts. Blanchard, for example, recorded in 1936 a case of reading and writing retardation in an eight-year old boy who had been placed in a foster-home by his mother. Whether the case was actually one of developmental dyslexia is not certain. The child's errors in writing were regarded by the analyst as signs of an underlying aggression towards his mother. In addition the boy indulged at times in meaningless scribbling which he spoke of as his "Chinese writing". To quote Blanchard . . . "he knew that the Chinese made peculiar marks to represent words: he had heard that the Chinese tortured people whom they hated". Blanchard went on to argue that the boy in his hatred towards his mother for deserting him felt like torturing her the way she had tortured him by securing his love and then rejecting him. His "Chinese writing" was, according to Blanchard, a magic spell that would cause his mother to be tortured with sharp knives or in other ways, and to be eaten by fierce animals.

Literary execution

Dyslexics, whatever their age, do not acquit themselves well in paper-and-pencil tests, though they may be able to express their ideas fluently by word of mouth. This discrepancy is more obvious in the older age-groups and in adult ex-dyslexics. A general slowness of writing has been emphasised earlier, but inadequacies in essay-writing are not due to this factor alone. Even when the writer is not working against the clock and has all the time he needs to construct and complete his essay or letter, the finished work may still show imperfections. These are manifold and can be traced to a number of different sources. One difficulty entails the correct use of punctuation, a problem which will be dealt with later.

When intelligent dyslexics have to sit formal examinations, they are often well aware of their particular shortcomings and their enhancement in such circumstances. The same girl of 15·09 years who is quoted on page 36 describing her difficulties of comprehension, went on to explain her problems with written work:–

> "*. . Then as time passes my hand writeing gets sluvenly and spellings become wrose. I am not sure where to use long words and when not to and I do not have a very wide vocabulary. My spelling is undiscribably bad and general layout of an essay is usually jumbled. Allthough I try to get a good content in my essays the result is usually jumbled and ilegibal*".

The written work of a dyslexic probably betrays evidence of a relatively small vocabulary. The longer the text, the more obvious this factor becomes. Up to a point, the limitation in words is realised by the dyslectic writer himself, who may try to avoid spelling mistakes by resorting to words which are simple and short. But such an explanation is not enough to account wholly for the meagre verbal repository. It could be argued that the young dyslexic may not have grown up in a bookish environment. From his simple reading-material he may not have acquired the storehouse of words which a good reader steadily and naturally assimilates. But other dyslexics come from cultured and educated families, and may have absorbed something from the richly worded conversation which he hears. If so he is fortunate, but the young dyslexic will still find it difficult to relate the sounds of some of the terms he hears with their visual appearances in print. A dyslexic from a lower social group may be underprivileged as regards the talk which goes on around him. To this detriment must be added the limited knowledge he absorbs from reading. Consequently when it comes to written composition, he is hindered by a paucity of words. This poverty applies both to the *available* vocabulary (made up of words which he understands but rarely employs), and to the *working* or *applied* vocabulary— which is the smaller stock of terms in daily usage.

A study of the letters and essays of a dyslexic, whatever his age, demonstrates the limited number of words which is utilized.

His spontaneous written work is brief compared with that of his peers of comparable age and intelligence, and the number of tokens (which is the technical expression used by linguists for the number of words in a text) is relatively few. An analysis of the tokens shows, moreover, that the writer is using few *different* words (or "types"). Some words appear again and again. To a linguist, a comparison between the types and tokens in an essay is significant, and this "T.T.R." or "type-token ratio" differs according to a writer's skill. Take for comparison two vastly different pieces of writing. First, the sentence "here is the beginning, here is the end; here is the way in, here is the way out", is made up of 18 tokens (or words); but because so many terms are repeated, the number of *different* words ("types") is nine. The type/token ratio is, therefore, 9 divided by 18, i.e. 0·5. By way of contrast, although "A boy stood on the burning deck when all but he had fled miles away fast and furiously" also comprises 18 tokens, no word appears more than once. Consequently there are 18 types and the type/token ratio is 1·0.

Both these sentences are relatively short. If one were to study longer pieces of prose, the prospect of a greater number of type-repetitions would increase, and there would be a less striking contrast in the T.T.R. than 0·5 as opposed to 1·0.

This fact is illustrated in two other texts, again very different in character. Let us compare two interesting pices of writing, the first by James Agate:

> "*I can recall a gate overlooking a rich vale, a sunset and some cows, and an older person telling me that one day these things would make me sad. Sometimes an odd view of the sea comes upon me, seen from an elevation of three feet or so—and suddenly I taste cold milk and have difficulty in putting on a pair of cream-coloured socks*".

The second text reads:

> "*Dear Mum and Dad and loving sisters, Rose, Mabel and our Gladys. I am very pleased to write you another welcome letter as this leaves me at present. Dear Mum and Dad and loving sisters, keep the home fires burning. Not 'arf. The boys are in the pink. Not 'arf. Dear loving sisters, Rose, Mabel and our Gladys, keep merry and bright, not 'arf*".

While there is no evidence that the latter was written by a

dyslexic, it is not straining credulity to suspect that, if genuine, it was the work of no scholar. This letter also appears in Agate's Memoirs, but it is not clear whether he himself wrote it, or, whether he merely quoted it. It could well be bogus —a literary leg-pull.

The two specimens are of equal length. Each is made up of 64 words, that is, 64 "tokens". Specimen (2), however, is highly repetitious, and the writer has made use of comparatively few *different* words or "types"; in fact, only 38. The type-token ratio is therefore, 0·59. In specimen (1), which is a polished and professional piece of writing, we find that the author has repeated himself scarcely at all. Twice he has used "I" and three times "me". The indefinite article appears seven times. This yields 61 "types" out of a total of 64 "tokens", giving a T.T.R. of 0·95.

Such differences are striking. Typically one finds a low T.T.R. in the writings of those who are immature, and it might also be observed in the work of a young dyslexic.

Quite apart from the richness or poverty of vocabulary, another index of literary immaturity is the meaning or "reference-function". The unknown letter-writer of specimen (2) has little or nothing to say. He gives a string of reiterations; five meaningless clichés, and on three occasions the verbal expletive "not 'arf". The whole letter is little more than a vague, groping attempt at communication, an uncouth *cri de coeur*.

In both written and spoken speech, each word, or more often a combination of words, which carries a definite idea or message, is technically spoken of as a "narreme", or unit of meaning. In specimen (2) there are only six or seven unconvincing "narremes". Specimen (1), however, is replete with meaning as well as various stimulating allusions. There are at least 14 "narremes" within the total of 64 words.

Narremic poverty is a feature which distinguishes the writings of a near-illiterate from those of a cultured and experienced author. To some extent this also applies in developmental dyslexia, for there is a correlation of a kind. Probably the all-important factor, however, is one of basic intelligence.

An example is the following first draft of an essay written by an intelligent dyslexic boy of 10·05 years, but the corrected version is not much better. The numerous erasures and corrections are not reproduced, and an interpretation of some of the more unusual neologisms is put within brackets.

"Hellow Maivis I prannownst, (?pronounced) can you get my house (horse) ready. Allright she replyed, weroe (where) are you ridding out, Today a new place Today, I think it is called Monks Wood, She turned round quickley droped the sadle. She was gave A startled look what iis the matter I said speak up, well that there Woddyg, haunted Haunted, yes Haunted, don't be danfed (daft) theres no such thing as ghosts. I wouldnt go in that wood for a Hundred pound". You arent serious are you as I mounted my horse and rode away down the wood. When I got there my horse hesitated for a minuete (minute) until I got my croup (crop) in action. We had Just gon a little way when I haerd (heard) a nois I looked round and saw ghast of a Monk. IT was coming towards us we started gallop away I was petrafied (petrified) a low branch noked (knocked me) off. I hit My head on a lange (?) and the everything was blanck. I woke up and found my self in Hospital".

This story is made up of 172 "tokens" or words. Of these, 102 are separate types. Therefore, in this essay the type-token ratio is 0·59, which corresponds exactly with the figure arrived at in the soldier's letter quoted by James Agate. This dyslexic resembles, therefore, the illiterate in his restricted vocabulary. When, however, we take note of the number of ideas that are expressed, we find that there are approximately 34 distinct "narremes" in the composition written by the dyslectic child. In the letter quoted earlier (specimen (2)) there were six "narremes" out of 64 words; in James Agate's own essay of the same length, at least 14. The dyslexic's story is nearly three times as long as both specimens (1) and (2). It might have been expected, therefore, that the two texts would yield 18 and 42 "narremes" respectively. The dyslectic boy is consequently shown to be less rich in ideas than James Agate, but significantly better than the writer of the second letter.

To take another example, the following is a transcription of a piece of spontaneous writing executed in about 20 minutes by a dullard, an adolescent much retarded as regards reading, spelling and numeracy. He was referred as a putative case of dyslexia.

"One day I went to car shop to look car at [a] car was [a] Renault 5LS and the men in the car shop was a Renault 5LS and the car had 8V cylinders and the had a red door and the men with a car look [ed] at the car and the car had a V8 cylinders and car the went [on] a car hill and the car went ar to [the] car shop and the boys went [to] see David dad car and the boys went home."

The words in brackets were omitted by the writer, and those

with an oblique line through them were corrections which he had made.

This text comprises 81 tokens, and the T/T ratio is as low as 0·24. The narremic value of his composition was possibly nine.

Expressed differently, we can say that James Agate took four words to express a concept; the dyslectic boy five words; the dullard nine words; and the soldier letter-writer 10·5.

Apart from straightforward encoding of information there exists another and very different side to a dyslexic's composition.

Many dyslectic boys and girls enjoy listening to poetry, and it has been an intriguing experience to find dyslexics who have ventured into creative versification, and who sometimes display no little talent. A few verses have even been published. One of the youngest from our series was a boy of 8·04 years who won a prize for the following poem entitled *Silver*:

> "*Silver is shiny,*
> *Silver is money,*
> *Silver shows that a man is rich,*
> *Silver is a shiny door.*
> *Silver is a young summer night,*
> *Silver is like a glittering eye in the dark.*
> *Silver is in a hare,*
> *Silver is in a tower.*
> *Silver is a peaceful light,*
> *Silver is a glittering sight.*
> *Silver is a moon so bright,*
> *Silver is a glittering heart,*
> *Silver is the rain,*
> *Silver is the bark on a tree,*
> *Silver is the happy year gone by,*
> *Silver is an old man's hair,*
> *Silver is a dog.*
> *Silver is a well-known man,*
> *Silver is living so sweet,*
> *Silver is a dewy morning,*
> *Silver is the grass on a sunny night.*"

From numerous other examples, the next was written by a dyslectic girl of 17, who confessed that at the time she had been deeply despondent.

> "*It is all for the best*
> ——————————————
> *Night, confusion, cold.*

All for the best.
Police, danger, hate, warmth,
happiness, freedom.
   All for the best.
Freedom to do more or less what I wanted to do
   It was all for the best.
Freedom of speech.
Does that not matter more? Yes.
But freedom of the mind matters most to me.
Capture freedom of the mind and go
on to capture freedom of speech.
How would you know that you have
captured freedom of the mind
Well it would be like hearing Billie
Holiday and going off to sleep and
waking up and hearing Billie singing.
It would be so beautiful
Words cannot explain
All I know is freedom of the mind would be it."

It may seem odd that dyslexics—who are typically reluctant and indifferent essayists—are able to express themselves in verse comparatively well, and furthermore take considerable pleasure in this art-form. Might it be that verse is an easier medium for one who is lame in his power of self-expression? This phenomenon has indeed also been found in some adults who become aphasic because of acquired brain-damage. One aphasiac successfully marketed a poem at a time when he could scarcely write a simple letter to his relative.

Why should verse be easier? It is interesting that George Meredith expressed this opinion one hundred years ago.

Below a certain level of attainment, poetry is less demanding than prose, especially if the verse is of the "free" type and therefore unhampered by considerations of metre, scansion, assonance or rhythm. In serious prose, each word chosen by the writer is the only one which wholly fits the context and which gives vent to what is in the writer's mind. The poet, however, may use quite simple and easily manipulated words. This is because the word chosen need not be precise, or constitute the veritable *mot juste*. It can be relatively vague, but allusive, evocative, stimulating, metaphorical. If too difficult to spell, that particular word can be bypassed. In writing verse, syntax can be jettisoned in a way which would be impossible for an essayist. Or it might be that the author's thinking is a little nebulous and ill-defined. If so, to versify would be the ideal method of expression and one which would bring the most pleasure to the writer.

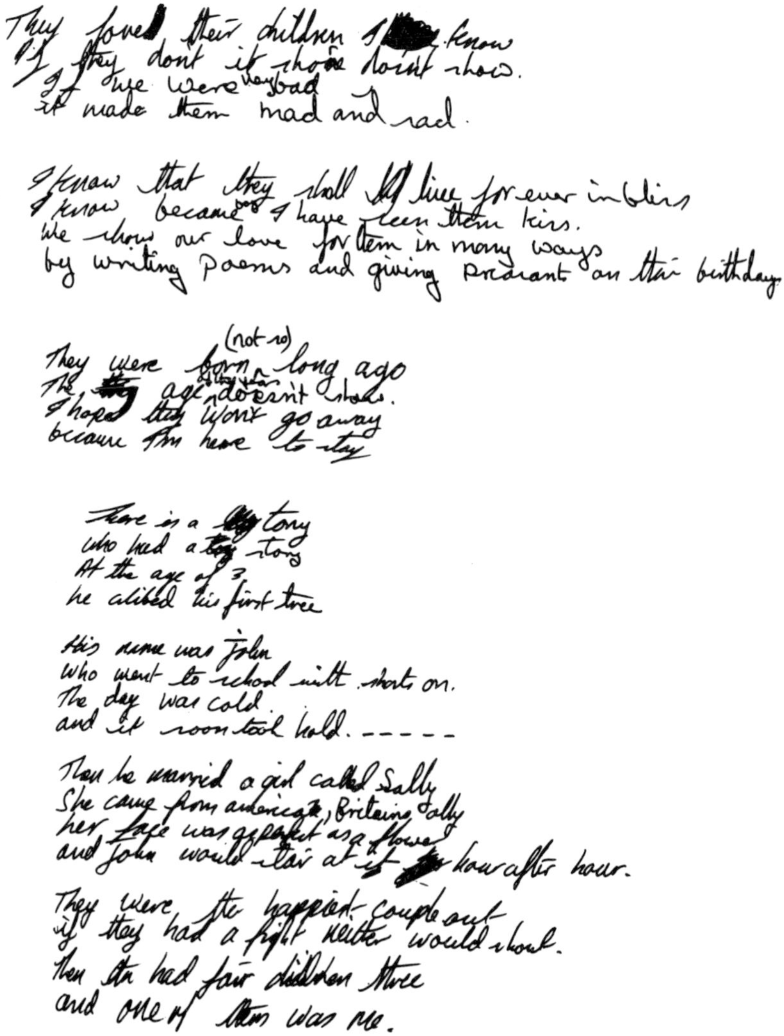

They loved their children I know
If they dont it shows doesnt show.
If we were they bad
it made them mad and sad.

I know that they shall live for ever in bliss
I know because I have seen them kiss.
We show our love for them in many ways
by writing poems and giving presants on their birthday

They were born (not so) long ago
The age doesnt show.
I hope they won't go away
because I'm here to stay

There is a tony
who had a story
At the age of 3
he climbed his first tree

His name was John
who went to school with shorts on.
The day was cold
and it soon took hold. -----

Then he married a girl called Sally
She came from america, Britains ally
her face was as perfect as a flower
and John would stair at it hour after hour.

They were the happiest couple out
if they had a fight neither would shout.
Then they had fair children three
and one of them was me.

Fig. 20 Poem written by a dyslectic boy of 15 years. (R.A. 14+; Sp.A. – 13).

To a dyslexic who happens to be sensitive and thoughtful as well as intelligent, verse has perhaps more to offer than prose. His creative imagery may be bursting to declare itself—in the spoken word if possible; if not, then in poetry rather than the arid precision which good prose-writing ordains.

Vers libre, therefore, is a suitable medium to link those outside the communicative network with the dyslexic who is within. If thoughts cannot be spoken, let them be sung.

One boy of 15·08 years, a resolving dyslexic of superior intelligence, expressed his creative abilities in "concrete" verse. An illustration of one of his calligrams is shown in Fig. 21.

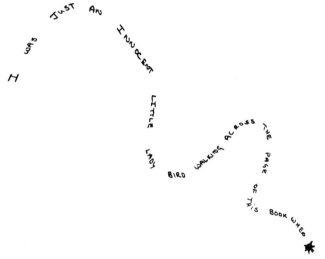

Fig. 21 Calligram written by a resolving dyslexic interested in abstract versification. Male, aged 15.08 (R.A. 14+; Sp.A. 13.06; IQ 135). The text reads: "I was just an innocent little ladybird walking across the page of this book when ✹."

Punctuation

When a dyslectic child writes an essay or letter, he is usually sparing in the use of punctuation marks. For example, in the following story of 158 words, penned by a boy with developmental dyslexia aged 7·08 (full-scale I.Q. 108; reading age less than seven and a spelling age below six), it will be noted that there is not one attempt at punctuation.

"The Runner Bean

*wust a pona tim there wes a Bunner Bean and the Bean ran evre day 4 mist
and suma day pep trid to cash it an They cood not cash it decos it wos to
Frst and they trid and trid a trid and they poot sum floows out when it cam
nen the floows it wood be bont on its hed and it wood be coos and this wort
but it got a way and it did not run eny mor by it did do sum exsisis in hoos
and it did tac up fun and wun day I hop I wll to to the moon and hav a good
looza rood and do sum ic sperimp and fid sum tras of small and fid if ther
is clall up ther".*

In the next essay, a dyslectic child of eight years, with a reading
age of just under seven and a spelling age of −6., has written 132
words before he inserts a full stop. It is interesting that in the
first line he has placed a comma between the numerals 25 and the
word "feet", presumably with the intention of expressing "25,000
feet".

"BEA

*We flow 25, feet of grad and my ear drums berst went we came to laed and
they was a bres and we came down on a staer kaese and then we went to a
place ware a men chat are prslboat and then we went to get the lugig and
then we had a bare wath a man chat and then we met up to geter and then we
loke a tase to the dondy and prst a man on a bots To day was are ferst day
hear and it was verry verey hot me and Jolect went to get some bast to day
and we went swiming vast day in the sea and I got wash out to sea for my
2 time and we go swiming for shals".*

Three questions arise. Why should a dyslexic use punctuation
marks so little? Which types of mark does he utilise, albeit
infrequently, and which does he avoid altogether?

According to the Oxford English Dictionary punctuation may
be defined as "the practice, art, method or system of inserting
points or "stops" to aid the sense, in writing or printing; division
into sentences, clauses, etc. by means of points or stops". Punctuation is, therefore, a "paralinguistic" activity which affords the
reader an "over-text" or additional meaning to what has been
written.

Punctuation is influenced by the dictates of fashion as well as by
personal prejudices and preferences. Not only are there right and
wrong ways but—more subtle still—there are elegancies and
inelegancies. It is a lexico-semantic signalling system peculiar to
written and printed language, and corresponds roughly with
pauses and tonal inflexions in spoken speech. The marks also

assist one to read aloud in a convincing fashion. Punctuation is a grammatical refinement acquired later than the art of writing. Mastery in the orthodox as well as the more stylistic manipulation of these marks may be attained unduly late, and indeed may always elude the novice or the ill-educated. Perfection may also constitute an obstacle to a foreigner, for there are racio-linguistic differences in the use of punctuation. Germans are lavish with their exclamation marks or "christers", and in their correspondence use them after the introductory Dear Sir!—like a stick in a hedge. The Spaniard is logical; and, mindful of a reader's dilemma, helps him by starting an interrogatory sentence with an up-ended question mark (¿) which tells him in advance how to modulate his voice. He is conventional in finishing with a similar mark, this time the other way up. In Spanish a mark of exclamation is placed both at the beginning and at the end of a word or phrase, and in modern Greek a question mark is expressed as a semi-colon (;) and the colon by an inverted full stop (·).

When the dyslexic begins to tackle the problem of punctuating his laboured writing, he probably first becomes proficient in the use of the full-stop. A tentative introduction of commas—never an easy task even to the initiated—comes much later. Inverted commas and brackets next appear, while question marks, colons, semi-colons, and dashes, trail far behind.

A punctuation-count can be made and applied to an essay written by a dyslexic and then compared with the writing of a non-dyslexic. But to determine with precision any differences that may appear, it is necessary to compare two texts which are identical as regards theme and choice of words.

A non-dyslexic might write something like:

> " "*My God!*", he said, "*what are you saying? The decision is difficult; the material comes in various shapes—square, oval, triangular. Then there is a choice of colours: brown, blue, green and so on. You will find everything you want at Simpsons' in St. James's Street.*"

Spelling-errors apart, a dyslexic might write the same text but punctuated erratically:

> "*My God he said, what are you saying. The decision is difficult, the material comes in various shapes square oval triangular Then there is a choice of colours, brown blue green and so on. You will find everything you want at Simpsons in St. Jame's Street*".

Two more examples of creative work by dyslexics are quoted in order to show the beginnings of the use of punctuation. The first is a poem written by a mild or "borderline" dyslexic girl of 8·11 years with a reading age of eight.

> " *The water flows*
> *The water folls down the water flows and*
> *make a luvly noise. It is the craching*
> *trees craching together.*
> *When it is witer it is all frozen up and*
> *children play on it skiding about. They*
> *fall over cwite a lot.*
> *When it is summer again all the children*
> *pot on a boat on a river and go for a ride.*
> *To see the wild flowers.*
> *The water flows fill happy want agan,*
> *The children should agan to see the petty*
> *water folls wants agan".*

The second comes from an interesting and thoughtful essay entitled "The Frustrations of Dyslexia". The writer was an intelligent girl aged 16·1 years, whose spelling age was ten.

> *"But I have been extremely lucky. And I am aware of the fact that I have escaped exceedingly lightly Also that if my parents had been less perspicatious, or if I had (lived) been born even 10 years earlier when the word was vertualy unknown the brand "lazy" would still be fresh and one of my greatest debts should be paied to such pioneers as my doctor".*

(The word in brackets had been erased by the writer herself.)

Copying

It is sometimes said that, whatever other mistakes he perpetrates, a dyslectic child makes no errors in copying a text set before him, for the task merely entails the execution of a faithful reproduction of what he sees.

This is not necessarily so; errors may occasionally creep in.

Should a very young child consistently make mistakes when copying from a blackboard, it is important in the first place that his vision be tested. Even when a child is known to be dyslexic, inaccuracies in copying may not be entirely the result of the underlying dyslexia. The dyslectic child could have a coincidental refractive error, which adds to his problems by preventing him from seeing clearly the words chalked on the blackboard.

It is important to realise the magnitude of the task which confronts any child who is learning to read and to write, and to understand why a young dyslexic fails to achieve a rapid mastery of these arts. He has to learn that the lower case "pig" means the same as the upper case "PIG", and, moreover, the same as *pig* in cursive. The first is what he encounters in a book, the next is in the title and the last has been written by his teacher. Here then are three different sets of symbols indicating the same idea.

This is bad enough, but the child must also learn that 𝒢𝒢𝑔ℊℊ are variant forms for what the teacher may have told him was a "gee" or a "gh"; and yet the sound "gh", although appropriate in the word "go", is wrong when it comes to reading the word "gym". The alphabet, he finds, is full of alternative forms, some appropriate for writing and others for print, some for reading aloud, and some for silent interpretation. 𝒯𝓉𝓉𝒯𝒯 are all acceptable. So are 𝒮𝓈𝓈𝓈. In other words, the learner has to cope with not a mere 26 letters of the alphabet, but perhaps four or five times as many different shapes as well. There is even another symbol—the ampersand.

Taking a minimum four variant forms for each individual letter, the child has to master 104 different signs quite apart from the ten numerals. In practice, the total figure approaches nearly 200 graphic marks.

If the young child has been subjected to the initial teaching alphabet technique of learning symbols, his task of transcription becomes still harder, and it may be a detriment to learning in the case of a dyslexic.

Furthermore, he may hear the letters enunciated in the conventional fashion *ay, bee, see, dee, ee, eff, gee*, and so on, while another teacher may use the "phonetic", *ah, buh, kuh, duh, e, ff*, etc. Most young readers try out their newly learned reading skill on streetsigns, hoardings, magazines, advertisements, as well as in books at home. In doing so, he comes up against a whole gamut of different "type-faces", some of them fairly common, like italic print, others extremely elaborate such as the outmoded blackletter style of printing (Gothic, *Fraktur*, or "old English"). A century ago, typography came under the influence of *art nouveau* which brought about even further liberties with the design of the letters of the alphabet. Purists were offended by some of the exuberancies which were regarded as vulgar, even indecent. In 1931 that master of calligraphy, Eric Gill, said:

"*. . . the business of printed lettering has now, under the spur of commercial competition, got altogether out of hand and gone mad. There are now about as many different varieties of letters as there are different kinds of fools. I myself am responsible for designing five different sorts of sans-serif letters—each one thicker and fatter than the last because every advertisement has to try and shout down its neighbours. And as there are a thousand different sorts of fancy lettering so there are many too many different sorts of type for reading in books—all of them copies and resuscitations and re-hashes and corruptions of the printing types designed for modern machine production; and the machines themselves are complicated by every sort of complicated mechanism for producing the appearance of pre-industrial things. You cannot put back the clock—no. But you can at least recognise that a certain amount of time has passed and not pretend that we are still ancient Britons*".

It follows, therefore, that when a child embarks upon the task of "copying" he does not merely make a slavish replica of a printed or written text. The problem goes deeper. Copying usually entails some measure of interpretation and this is a double—if not a three-fold exercise in cognition. The child sees in his book the word *donkey* or perhaps *DONKEY*, but before he realises that the two symbols have the same meaning, he must first surmount a process of identification. This procedure usually comprises a recognition of the constituent letters, and then the extraction of meaning. The second part is not essential, for a child might be able to transcribe faithfully but not know what the combination of letters means. After this two-fold operation, he must recall the appropriate graphic marks before he can commit the word to paper. Understanding these cognitive processes helps to explain why a young dyslexic may make mistakes in copying.

An interesting type of mistake was observed when one young dyslexic was told to practise writing by copying a series of two "joined-up" letters, such as *be*, *by*, *do*, *go* and *he*. He consistently wrote the word *be* with the vowel inverted in the following way: *be*. All the other two-letter words were, however, copied correctly.

Another cause of error in copying stems from a hurried "flash" identification of a word. This is most likely to occur in the case of "homophones", or words which sound alike but differ in meaning. Thus a dyslectic child may identify the word "there" as a whole, realise how it sounds when spoken, but then write it down as "their".

Ordinarily any child of about eight years can be expected to have mastered successfully the conversion of Roman print into flowing handscript. As a routine test, a child aged 13 years or under is asked to copy as much as possible from a printed text in precisely 60 seconds and to write as quickly as he can. The model is printed in Roman lower case letters, and the child makes his copy in traditional cursive, "joined-up" writing. The rate of writing is measured by counting the number of letters written during the 60 seconds, and recorded as the G.U.S. (graphic units per second) ratio as described in Chapter 4. The morphology of the penmanship should be noted, particularly the size of the middle zone letters; the formation of the individual characters; the number of erasures; and the spacing between consecutive letters. In other words, a superficial examination of the penmanship should be made along the lines described in Chapter 4. Lastly one scrutinizes the writing for faults in copying, that is, mis-spellings, omission of letters or of whole words, or repetition of letters, syllables or words.

It may be argued that in copying, a child is influenced—helped perhaps, possibly hindered—by the fact that as he writes he may simultaneously be engaged in interpreting the *meaning* of what he copies. This possibility can be investigated by next getting him to copy a series of nonsense-phrases, or else a text printed in a language foreign to him. The child is asked to reproduce it as quickly as possible in his usual cursive script, from a model which is printed in upper case lettering.

Again he writes as fast as he can for 60 seconds, and is then stopped even if he has to leave a word unfinished. The same features are recorded; the number of "characters"; the number of errors; and the nature of the penmanship.

In our series of 444 patients, with only one exception, the results were much the same in both tests. The errors were neither more nor less, and the sum-total of letters transcribed in 60 seconds was roughly the same. The principal difference lay in the nature of the child's handwriting, suggesting that his main difficulty was not in copying but in the conversion of capital letters into cursive. Many dyslexics reproduce the upper case type, though they have been specifically instructed not to do so. Older dyslexics may continue to confuse upper and lower cases when copying and interpolate capital letters within the body of their cursive writing now and again.

In the case of a dyslexic who is about 13 years of age or more, the test of copying is presented in a different way. He is confronted with a text of 113 simple words, no one of which is "difficult", polysyllabic or likely to be unfamiliar, and he is asked to copy it as quickly as possible. This task can be effected by a non-dyslexic in $2\frac{1}{2}$ to 3 minutes. Dyslexics and most ex-dyslexics are far slower, and sometimes errors in spelling and also omission of words may be observed. Sometimes, too, the writer finds he has written a phrase twice and crosses out the unwanted repetition. He may explain such a mistake by saying that he had difficulty in "finding his place" when reading the model.

Spelling

In considering a young dyslexic's troubles, it is all too easy to focus attention exclusively upon his difficulties in learning to read. The task of writing which later confronts him will constitute even more of an obstacle, and the first impediment to be overcome is spelling. The English language, like French and Erse, is notorious for its illogical spelling. Many years ago, at least one writer seriously suggested that dyslexia was a condition peculiar to English-speaking children. Experience has since discounted this idea, and we now have good reason to believe that no race escapes its quota of late, inaccurate, or poor readers, some of whom may well be examples of developmental dyslexia.

To say this is not to overlook the fact that a young English-speaking child faces a greater obstacle in learning to read his mother tongue than, say, an Italian, whose language is comfortably rational as regards its orthography. The following lines illustrate the pitfalls which confront the English-speaking child:

> "*Though from rough cough and hiccough free,*
>   *That man has pain enough,*
> *Whose wounds, plough through, sunk in a slough*
>   *Or lough, begin to slough*".

Before discussing the dyslexic's difficulty in spelling, one must take into consideration the fact that in recent years accuracy of spelling generally is not considered as important as it was two or three generations ago. Even in academic and professional circles standards of spelling, like handwriting, have slipped. Dr. Meyer, the founder of Millfield School, in a personal communication wrote. "I have known a boy getting good passes in what at times he calls "Physcics," "Chesmistry" and "Boilogy". I have also known an "A" level English Literature candidate who got away with essays on "Dicksen", "Kaets" and "Bryon" . . ." These were not dyslectic boys, be it added. One of us has had the experience of marking M.D. theses, and in three out of four of them the candidate wrote "Medecine" at the head of his essay. The low level of contemporary spelling has been the subject of a Governmental paper and numerous letters have appeared in the correspondence columns of the Press. To some degree the situation is reminiscent of what obtained in the time of Chaucer, Shakespeare and even throughout the 17th century. At a meeting of the British Association in 1976, Dr. Uta Frith drew attention to a number of intelligent pupils who were good readers but poor spellers. "In this sense", she said, "we must conclude that reading and writing a word correctly do belong together. Ideally they should be two sides of the same coin, but this study has shown that this is not a necessary state of affairs".

Being, as W. S. Gilbert put it, "shaky in his spelling", the dyslexic will suffer from this particular handicap more severely and will wrestle with it for longer than it will take him to master the art of reading. Thus, when there is typically a gap of two years between the chronological and the reading ages, the spelling age might well trail four years behind the actual age. Even when the adolescent or adult dyslexic is reading with enjoyment, in all likelihood he will still be an unsound and inconsistent speller.

There seems to be only one reference in the world's literature to poor readers who are better spellers. In Uruguay 118 third-grade schoolchildren were tested. 31 (or 26%) were found to be poor readers but they could spell better than they could read. The writer, Carbonell de Grampone (1974), estimated that members of this group had good auditory perception but difficulties in visual perception, and related this fact to the structure of the Spanish language.

An older dyslexic often finds that his writing, though not his speech, is halting. He may have doubts about the spelling of the word that he would like to use. His pen is arrested while he searches in his mind for synonyms or circumlocutions that are both satisfying and within his ability to spell.

One characteristic feature of the spelling of a dyslexic is its inconsistency. A word might be spelled correctly in one place, but quite differently a little later. Indeed, within a single paragraph a word may appear in four or five different versions.

In relatively young dyslexics, the ability to spell aloud may differ from the ability to spell on paper. As a rule the former is more accurate.

When in doubt as to the precise spelling of a word, most people are able to write down the alternatives and choose the correct version, but dyslexics do not have this ability. Often they cannot detect mistakes perpetrated by themselves or by others, whether in print or handwriting. Professional sign-writers have been known to be oblivious of faults in their spelling, and one has encountered such street-signs as *SOLW* (slow); *TAIS*(taxis); *HOSIPTAL* (hospital); *OLNY* (only); *AHⱯAD* (ahead); and *SLOW TURCKS* (slow trucks). When dyslexics are confronted by a photograph of such words, they scarcely ever detect the error.

Despite their diversity, the mis-spellings commonly perpetrated by dyslexics can be analysed. The chief errors may be classified as follows:

Phonetic Substitution. This is perhaps the commonest, and it indicates an inability to overcome the orthographic inconsistencies of the English language. The writer correlates sound with appearance in a logical, but incorrect fashion. Hence, *kof, plow, cum, pikchur,* for *cough, plough, come, picture,* do at least suggest that the dyslexic's auditory processing is intact. Phonetic mistakes of this kind do not necessarily mar the intelligibility of their written work. This defect, of course, is not confined to developmental dyslexics.

Dyslexics also find it difficult to distinguish homophonic words, that is, those which sound alike but differ in both meaning and spelling. Thus, *flour* and *flower* may be used by them interchangeably. Similarly *rite* and *right, so* and *sew, their* and *there, wear, where* or *were.*

Approximate Phonetic Substitutions. These are the dyslexic's mis-spellings which only partly resemble the sound, e.g. *toch* (for *took*); *bicos* (for *because*); *done* (for *down*); *orll* (for *all*); *alfnt* for *elephant.* The differences usually concern the vowels, but when a dyslexic writes *cot* instead of *got, dit* instead of *bit, dat* for *bat,* the error lies in a confusion of similar sounding consonants. This is rarer, and raises the possibility of an associated "dysphonemia" or an inability to distinguish by ear, sounds which are closely related.

Rotations and Reversals. These are common dyslectic errors. Rotation means a letter which is incorrectly orientated in its lateral dimension. Commonest among such rotations are *d* for *b*, *b* for *d*. Hence it is not unusual for a dyslexic to write *bog, bab, done, dut*, instead of *dog, dad, bone, but*. In such cases interpretation is not always easy; even the dyslexic himself, after an interval of time, may be at a loss to read back what he had written earlier and make sense of it. Up-down reversals are much rarer, but they sometimes appear, as shown by a confusion between *h* and *y*, so that occasionally *yat, yid, yim*, are written instead of *hat, hid, him*, or *hes, hell, hon*, for *yes, yell, yon*.

The term reversal is used when groups of two or more letters are written backwards, each individual letter being correctly orientated. This type of error occurs almost as often as a rotation of an isolated letter. It is common to find a dyslexic writing *tac* for *cat*, although he may write *cat* later in the same essay. *Form* for *from* and *carsh* for *crash* are examples of "inner" reversals; "held" may be written correctly in one place and appear as *hedl* or *hled* later on the same page.

"Mirror-writing" is the term used when each individual character is rotated and the order of the letters in a word is also reversed. Such writing can be deciphered if it is held in front of a

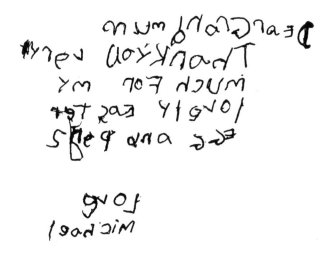

Fig. 22 Mirror-writing executed in the spontaneous work of a boy aged 5.06 years, who, when seen again at the age of 11.04 years was dyslexic. (R.A. 7.06; Sp.A. 7.06).

looking glass, or if the sheet of paper is turned round, held up to the light, and viewed from behind. Mirror-writing is never printed but only occurs in flowing handwriting. It is only perpetrated by some young left-handed dyslexics. Examples of mirror-writing are ᴄᴀᴛ for *cat* and ᴅᴏɢ for *dog*.

Omission of letters. This is common and can be seen when the dyslexic shortens his words by substituting, say, a single for a double letter; e.g. *shal, holow, to, mery, Jimy,* instead of *shall, hollow, too, merry, Jimmy,* and *atacking* for *attacking.* Another type of mistake is the omission of one letter or more from the body of a word, e.g. *ral (rail)*; *rember (remember)*; *tring (trying)*.

More complicated faults are exemplified in *iei* (for *river*); *sap* (for *camping*); *asmand* for *island.* Such mysterious transformations are not unusual in the writings of a very young dyslexic.

Confused Serialisation. Here all the appropriate letters are used but in a jumbled order, not explicable on the basis of rotations and inner reversals. Thus the dyslexic may want to write *stopped*, but he produces on paper *sdoptep*. Or, instead of *pencil*, he may write *plncie.* In most cases of defective serial order in spelling, the writer chooses the correct initial letter, but muddles the others.

The reason for confused serialisation lies at a deep cognitive level. On specific testing it will usually be found that the patient has only a hazy visual image of the precise order of the individual letters of the alphabet. The first few letters, perhaps as far as G, may be established firmly enough, but beyond that point he gets mixed up except possibly for accurate brief runs or "chunks" such as l-m-n, or p-q-r-s. Inaccurate sequencing can be uncovered by asking "which comes first: *t* or *q*?" Many—perhaps most—dyslexics hesitate before answering. Some reply immediately but incorrectly. Often the child moves his lips inaudibly, indicating that he is rapidly running through the alphabet from the beginning.

Confusion as to the serial order of the letters of the alphabet leads to other difficulties when the dyslexic is older. He is slow in looking up the correct spelling of an unfamiliar word in a dictionary, his eye not being able logically and rapidly to light upon the one that is wanted. Nor can he consult an index with speed and confidence. Even greater difficulty is entailed in coping with a telephone directory. As a routine test many patients in our series were told to look up the number in the London telephone directory of "J. M. McDonald". An intelligent non-dyslectic adolescent can usually do this within thirty seconds; however, a dyslexic may take ten minutes or more before he finds the required name and number.

In later life dyslexics employed in offices are inefficient at filing, for they cannot put documents away in the appropriate alphabetical order. This fault may be discovered by other workers in the office, rather than by the individual concerned, who simply reports that the required paper "is missing" when asked to produce a file that he or she has previously stored.

Of particular interest is the fact that this inherent defect in serialisation is not confined to letters of the alphabet. It also applies to the months of the year, so that a dyslexic may be unable quickly to state which is the fifth month, or the ninth. Again in his efforts to reply, the dyslexic may be observed to move his lips and his fingers in the process of quietly saying to himself "January, February, March . . ." and so on. Historical personalities and past events are likewise confused in time. Thus it is not easy for the dyslectic schoolboy to memorize the succession of the British monarchs, or prime ministers. In isolation, however, this defect may also apply to non-dyslexics.

Something comparable occurs with arithmetic. Many dyslexics, whether or not they happen also to show difficulties with numeracy, are late in memorising their "tables", because this represents an inherent problem in retaining and retrieving a complex load of information.

Dyslexics of an older age and also "ex-dyslexics" may be able to answer the question whether or not they possess a keen imagery of a number-form. This means the visualisation of the numbers one to 100, or perhaps the months of the year or the days of the week, as being arranged in a fixed and idiosyncratic pattern, such as, for example, a circle or an oval, or a straight line running from left to right either horizontal or tilted. Sometimes the arrangement is like the jagged formation of a graph, with peaks and valleys. The pattern is always highly personal, but relatively few, however, are endowed in this way.

Because of his difficulties with sequencing, a dyslexic might be expected not to be endowed with a number-form at all, or perhaps one which is unusual in character. A sensitive, intelligent ex-dyslectic girl of 19 was introspective enough to be able to describe her mental picture of the months of the year. She said they seemed to her to stretch along a very thin line, the middle parts being obscured by a fog-like blur, a kind of central scotoma within her visual imagery.

Superfluity of letters. A fault that a dyslexic may show is to lengthen a word by inappropriately adding syllables or letters. This defect is rather uncommon, however, except in simple words, such as *egge* for *egg*, *lowde* for *loud*, *worrie* for *worry*. They might be looked upon as phonetic substitutions, but the superfluous letters are often unexpected and apparently so illogical that the whole word becomes distorted. Other examples encountered in a random scrutiny of seven or eight essays are *toled*, *gardenning*, *payed*, *prarnowhst* (pronounced), *complently*, *plateform*, *woberli*, *gudenires* (gestures), *woulves*, *mornning*, *sulke*, *preasent*, *sparkelers*, *thinges*, *tolded*, *untill*, *writeing*, *birthaday*, *classe*, *colded*, *happerning*. This rather rare type of mis-spelling was referred to by Dickens in *Bleak House*:

> *"Caddy told me that her lover's education had been so neglected that it was not always easy to read his notes. She said if he were not so anxious about his spelling, and took less pains to make it clear, he would do better, but he puts so many unnecessary letters into short words, that they sometimes quite lost their English appearance."*

On the whole the tendency, however, is to shorten words. Examples of abbreviated words include *coed* (conquered), *lev* (leaving), *elvs* (elephants), *wen* (when), *midle* (middle), *richd* (reached), *tlvein* (television).

Bizarre spelling: This expression is commonly used in the literature on dyslexia. Some writers have said that many of the spelling mistakes made by a dyslexic can be described only by calling them "bizarre". Such a statement stresses the fact that a dyslexic's writings, whether spontaneous or to dictation, are quite unlike the faulty efforts of one whose education has been inadequate. Moreover, the mistakes are not always explicable along the lines already described, e.g. phonetic errors, defective serialisation, omissions, reduplications, and reversals. Sometimes no logical pattern can be discerned in the substitute word, and little or no relationship seems to exist between what the writer had in mind and what he puts down on paper. When such oddities abound, the text may be incomprehensible.

Examples of such "neographisms" or nonsense-words perpetrated by some dyslexics in our series are *aschle* (essential); *acdenter* (accidents); *satey* (safety); *ean* (end); *youy* (why); *Adto Fs*

(Arc de Triomphe); and *expectle* (especially). Only in some instances is the initial letter not that of the intended word. The most extreme example of dyslectic jargon-writing we have seen was all the more striking because the boy's penmanship was so clear that the errors were highlighted. The dyslexic, a boy of 10·08 years with a reading age of less than 6·06, had been told to take down the following piece of dictation, (a task obviously far beyond his capacity):

> "*Little Poppet lived in a house in the country with her Mummy and Daddy, her little brother and a shaggy dog called Timmy.*
> "*I am afraid I can't tell you what Little Poppet's real name was because I don't know, but as everyone always called her Little Poppet it doesn't really matter. Her little brother's name was Philip but he was always called Pip.*
> "*One morning Little Poppet and Pip went to do the shopping.*
> "*Wuff! Wuff! said Timmy. "I want to come too!"*
> "*Very well*", *said Little Poppet*, "*but you must keep close to us and not run off the pavement*".

The result was as follows, and the reader might well get the impression that he is looking at a foreign language or a meaningless cipher:

> "*In the pate leat tamey,*
> *lelat tomay (leal) yomly*
> *Hoyl Sah Mummy and Dad*
> *dy, Sah leat Sayh and*
> *theat leat gou hatay*
> *shapt.*
> *I hpeta a late I hglty ghat*
> *you onto leat haly*
> *gha holi reas Bhea het*
> *Heat I hgit ontgy Bgly*
> *thirat leayle Sah lact pat*
> *in Sakayg hgly yhegt.*
>
> *Sah yalaj Sgt ulas fat*
> *teat Bagleg Sgheaj ulas*
> *Salat hat trat.*
> *Are halej lyleg hat*
> *ylan and hayhe hfail*
> *ta hafgt fait leater.*
> *gooy gooy sglt laylea*
> *I ontg to hay to*
> *halgt Blajt you haly*
> *hghe hlglt to isdat*
> *and lalgt run hata*
> *falay hdgh.*"

It will be seen that strange and little used consonantal couplings recur. One wonders whether this may not be an example of what is referred to in this chapter on page 57 as "pentecostal" or "make-believe" writing. Here and there a pattern of error seems to be traceable as if representing a cipher. Malformation of some letters may have accounted for some mistakes in interpretation. Thus the recurring upper case "S" might actually have represented a lower case "h" written in an unorthodox way. The writer also made "t" and "l" look so alike that at times it was not easy to determine which letter was intended. This shows itself in the pseudo-words *laet, leat, leal, teat*. The looping of the upstroke often suggested an "l", and yet at times the symbol is both crossed and looped and may perhaps after all represent a "t".

It was interesting that the child could not subsequently read back a single word he had written; neither could his father, who had dictated the text to him.

Influence of distorted auditory input upon the ability to spell. Children learn to read not only by interpreting visual "graphemes", but also by correlating graphic marks with what they hear. There is a possibility that a teacher's diction might exert an influence upon the pupil's spelling if he possesses an emphatic regional accent with distorted vowel-sounds. The pupil may become relatively confused, and correlation between the sound and the verbal symbol may thus be strained; more so if the teacher's manner of speech differs from that of the child and his parents. It may also apply to a child born of immigrant parents, who hears one pattern of auditory symbols at home and another at school. Perceptual clashes engendered in this way are likely to aggravate any uncertainty in spelling on the part of the retarded reader but they are not its cause. The deleterious effect of the adult's diction on the child who is learning to talk, read and write, is surprisingly slight.

Chapter Five

Pre-dyslexia

"I never read much; I have something else to do".

Jane Austen

"Reading is seeing, by proxy".

Herbert Spencer

In Great Britain, where compulsory schooling starts at the age of five, a doctor will find it difficult to make a firm diagnosis of specific developmental dyslexia in a child under the age of seven years. Younger children have not been at school long enough for it to be certain that this is the explanation of an unexpected delay in learning to read. Nonetheless, in certain circumstances it may be possible to suspect that a child who is only six or even five years old will eventually prove to be dyslexic. The hybrid term "pre-dyslexia", though stylistically inelegant, indicates that there is an anticipatory stage which gives warning of future educational problems.

In the literature, many articles have dealt with early diagnosis. The writers do not necessarily mean "developmental dyslexia", but often assemble all children who have learning disabilities, whatever the cause. This lack of differentiation is unfortunate. The educational system in Great Britain differs from that which obtains in some other countries. Attendance at school is obligatory so that illiteracy resulting from lack of opportunity does not, or should not, occur. In the second place, schooling starts relatively early. Sometimes, indeed, the child will have been taught the letters of the alphabet by an attentive mother even in his pre-school days.

As stated in Chapter 3, some educationalists speak of "reading readiness". Presumably they have in mind a state of receptivity on the part of a child, indicating that he is ripe for instruction. This stage seems to be late in a child who subsequently shows the symptoms of developmental dyslexia.

Compulsory education starting at an early age means that the arts of reading and writing are instilled in circumstances which are potentially favourable. Hence the suspicion of an incipient reading-problem usually arises in the mind of the first teacher. Typically the child has reached and passed his developmental milestones at the appropriate times, that is, he has learned to walk and to talk at the usual age. He gives every indication at home of being bright, alert and alive to his environment. His memory is excellent, and his contacts with other children have always been good. Such is the opinion of the parents and grandparents and one which is shared at first by the teacher. It is, therefore, a matter of surprise when the child fails to keep up with others of the same age and comparable intelligence, and after a year or so he has trailed further behind.

In ideal circumstances the teacher informs the parents. If they are wise they will seek medical advice. The next step is careful testing of vision and hearing, for if the child needs glasses, or if he does not hear as well as he should, his educational progress may suffer. A child may fail to identify letters merely because he cannot perceive distinctly the writing on the blackboard. Or, should he not accurately hear the words spoken by the teacher, he will naturally find it difficult to correlate the sounds with the shapes of individual letters.

This initial stage of learning was familiar to Somerset Maugham, perhaps because of his medical training. In "The Verger" he wrote . . . "The cook tried to teach me to read, but I didn't seem to get the knack of it. I couldn't seem able to get the letters in me head when I was a nipper".

Still at this early stage of learning the alphabet, subtle unexpected features are apparent to the careful observer. The way the child handles cut-out letters may be revealing. The watchful onlooker may notice that the child is not only slow at identifying isolated letters, but the recognition of some of them presents more difficulty than others. Among the readily identified symbols are the vowels "o" and "i". Despite its infrequency, the symbol "x" is also usually grasped with comparative ease. Other letters present varying degrees of perceptual difficulty. Roughly speaking, the more elaborate the pattern of the letter, the easier the task. (This is quite unlike what occurs in a blind adult who is struggling to learn Braille with his finger-tips.) Thus "E" is often identified by a sighted child before "F", and "L" is recognised later still. The converse occurs in one who is bereft of sight. Still more important in the prediction of dyslexia, is a child's perceptual doubt as to the correct placement or positioning of letters in space. Most often this confusion applies to those letters that are asymmetrical in shape, e.g. "E", "F", "J", "K", "L", "P", "B". Of course, this phenomenon is not uncommon in young children who are not dyslexic, but their stage of doubt is shorter and disappears without leaving any further problems. Older ill-educated persons, not necessarily dyslexic, may also continue throughout life to perpetrate such errors as "и" for "N" and "Ƨ" for "S", though this is seen less often nowadays than it used to be.

Up-down confusion is particularly important, for it is not met within normal circumstances. Thus the pre-dyslexic may be in doubt as to the correct vertical disposition of some letters and numerals, causing him to write "Ⅎ" for "F", "Ꞁ" for "L", "ſ" for "J", "ᘔ" for "2". Moreover, when he is shown a cut-out letter that is incorrectly orientated, he might fail to detect the mistake.

At this point, mention should be made again of that interesting phenomenon of concretisation of literal symbols already touched upon in Chapter 3, even though it is uncertain whether it relates to the delay in learning to read. Sometimes it does and sometimes it does not, so perhaps it is no more than an epiphenomenon. Indeed, we are not even aware how common it is. Much of what is known results from the retrospective recollection of certain writers who are unlikely to have been victims of developmental dyslexia. The terms "literal concretisation" or "objectivation" refer to that trick of imagery whereby the young reader endows each letter of the alphabet with a simple mental association outside its usual function. As stated elsewhere in this book, "X" may be described by a child as a St. Andrew's Cross, or the letter "O" as a circle or a ball, or a "U" as a magnet, or an "I" as a pole.

Several examples of literal concretisation have also been quoted. Charles Dickens—anything but dyslexic himself—was a close observer of difficulties in reading in others, as shown by many passages in his novels. In *Great Expectations*, young Pip in his early efforts to read, identified an upper case "D" with a large buckle. In *David Copperfield*, Dickens wrote, "I thought the letters were printed and set there to plague me, and I look upon the printer as my greatest enemy. I never now see a row of large, fat, black, staring Roman capitals, but this reminiscence rises before me". G. K. Chesterton, an indifferent scholar in his early days, later recalled how his boyhood imagination had been arrested by the upper case letters of the Greek alphabet. To him *Theta* was a sphere girded around the middle like Saturn, and *Upsilon* was full of charm and mystery to him, for it stood erect like a chalice, tall and curved. On the other hand, the lower case Greek letters were nothing more than a series of "nasty little things like a swarm of gnats".

Such a phenomenon as concretisation of letters could not fail to intrigue psychologists interested in reading-problems. Faust (1954) referred to a patient with congenital *Schreib-Lese-Schwäche* (writing and reading weakness) to whom a capital "X" suggested a sawing trestle. To the same boy, a capital "Y" was a pole-support; an "S" a traffic sign; and a capital "P" either police or a post office. A capital "U" was a rounded arc, and "G" was an arc with a funny dash in it. Some psycho-analysts who have been bold enough to fish in these troubled waters characteristically retrieved flotsam and jetsam which were meaningful—to themselves at least. Thus Klein (1949) believed that the shape, appearance and even the sound of some letters might delay the acquisition of reading- and writing-skills by evoking distracting fantasies—oral, genital or urinary. Blanchard referred to a young child who was backward in his reading because, he said, he always associated the letter "C" with an open mouth ready to bite him.

Objectivation may apply to words as well as letters. For example, in an essay by a highly intelligent and articulate ex-dyslexic in which she described her earlier frustrations, she wrote (her own spelling is retained):

> "*When I was five the word "school" was abroaded in glories dreams coungered up with the aid of books to me. The dream and mistery was all too soon shattered . . the worst aspect was being a figure of fun. When amusement was wanted I'd have to write my name on the board. The result was a collection of letters that looked as if they had been saviarly tourtured. They were knarled and twisted like old and deformed people and turned upside down and inside out.*"

It might be thought that the habit of objectivation or con-cretising in a child who is learning to read would retard his progress by delaying recognition of the abstract properties of each letter. This is not borne out by the experience of Lady Diana Manners who wrote: "I learned that "E" was like a little carriage with a little seat for the driver and that "G" looked like a monkey eating a cake". She went on to say that her nannie taught her the letters on building-bricks and that she "learned to read without tears by the ripe age of four".

Another odd phenomenon which should alert attention and raise the suspicion that a pre-school child may eventually be late in learning to read, is the occasional practice of looking at picture-books upside down. In his scribbling and in his earliest efforts at drawing, he may also make sketches which are inverted. Up-down spatial confusion is unusual, and when it occurs an attentive parent usually notices it. A variant of this phenomenon, however, may appear later and escape observation. The child might draw a man standing the right way up but he starts with the feet and then proceeds to the legs, trunk and, last of all, to the head. This is common in young dyslectic patients, but whether more often than in non-dyslexics of the same age has yet to be substantiated.

The parents of some children who have later been established as developmental dyslexics have described other disorders of spatial thinking that were striking at the age of four or five years. The condition shows itself before the age at which the child can be expected to discriminate between right and left, and also before the identification of letters. He is muddled when confronted with ideas or commands which entail propositions of place or of time. He may not understand the distinction between up and down, or inside and outside. Moreover future and past tenses may be confused so that he is hazy as to the precise difference between soon and later, yesterday and tomorrow, finished and more to come. In concrete terms, the youngster may confound the bonnet of the car with the boot, the front garden with the back, upstairs and downstairs, the front from the back door, the attic of the house and the cellar.

Another characteristic sometimes displayed by the pre-dyslexic which may be predictive, is difficulty in copying from a blackboard or from a book. In Chapter 4 this topic was discussed, and the difficulties inherent in the act of copying were fully explained.

Among the formal studies dealing with the early forewarning of reading problems, McLeod (1966) spoke of a "predictive index".

However, it is in fact a scheme for the identification of a case which is already one of unequivocal dyslexia rather than a pre-dyslexia. Tower (1973) and Jansky (1973) are among the authors who have written upon this subject. The most comprehensive study, however, has been that of de Hirsch (1962–1965) in collaboration with Jansky and Langford. These authors listed some clinical features, which, in their opinion, when added to the results of special psychological test-procedures, constituted predictive signs of dyslexia. They mentioned small stature; over-activity (less often under-activity); limited span of auditory memory; distractability; impulsiveness; babyish behaviour; and ready fatigue. Comment on this study appears in *The Dyslexic Child*. M. Critchley (1970).

A fairly recent Americo-Australian research project seems to show that shrewd prediction is possible at the age of five, and before schooling has started. Professor Satz in 1970 tested 497 children who were unselected except for the fact that they constituted the entire white five-year old male population of Alachua County, Florida. Unfortunately details of his tests were not given, but he demarcated four groups, viz: (1) severe reading risk; (2) mild reading risk; (3) potentially average reader; and (4) potentially superior reader. The numbers falling into each group were not stated. These children were re-examined in 1973, that is, when they were in Grade II, and their reading ability assessed. It was found that a correct forecast has been made in 91 per cent of the boys in group (1); in 65 per cent of those in group (2); in 68 per cent in group (3); and 97 per cent in group (4).

Three years later, in 1976, 442 of the original 497 boys were still available for testing when they had reached Grade V. The original prognostication was found to have been correct in 58 per cent of those in group (1); in 20 per cent of those in group (2); 94 per cent of those in group (3) (i.e. "average"); and 99 per cent of those in group (4) (i.e. "superior"). The number of children with a reading disability had increased from 12 per cent in 1973 to 20 per cent in 1976. Had it been decided to initiate remedial treatment in 1970 on all the children placed within groups (1) and (2), the decision would have been justified in 88 per cent of the cases. Professor Satz stressed that the *research showed that the ingredients of reading failure are present in children before they enter school and are not the result of bad teaching by the classroom teacher.*

A personal communication from the Secretary of the Dyslexia Research Foundation of West Perth, Australia, indicates that Professor Satz's full data will soon be published.

Much of what has been written about hearald signs and symptoms should be treated with caution. Of necessity, the children under observation have been young, i.e. only four, five or six years of age. Records of behaviour, coupled with an exhaustive medical examination of the nervous system may have brought to light features which some authors regarded as anomalous. Whether any firm connection exists between these findings and the subsequent emergence of developmental dyslexia is uncertain. The suspicious signs may in fact have been little more than hallmarks of immaturity which steadily lessen and finally disappear as the child grows older. If, however, this is not the case, and these features persist after the age of seven or eight, then quite correctly the inkling grows that some organic, albeit mild structural or physiological, fault is present, but this may be something quite different from developmental dyslexia. In such cases there may be an associated learning disability and it should not necessarily be assumed to be specific developmental dyslexia, nor, in retrospect, would it have been correct to regard the earlier signs as having been portentous.

There is, however, one question which can be answered only by a combination of experience, sagacity and judgement on the part of a doctor. If we are right in regarding specific developmental dyslexia as a manifestation of belated cerebral maturation, then it would not be surprising if the dyslexic of seven years or so should, for a time, display other marks of immaturity. It is then necessary to decide whether they are indicative of developmental dyslexia, or whether they imply something else. At what age should they disappear in a non-dyslectic child? A longitudinal study comprising repeated clinical examinations together with careful assessments of scholastic achievement over a period of years, ought to answer this question.

Most attempts to presage developmental dyslexia have become unduly complicated, and it might be well to cut away some of the dead wood and declare a few simple propositions:

1. If an older sibling, or even a close relative, is known to be a genuine victim of developmental dyslexia, then the probability of a similar condition is high in a young child if signs of cerebral immaturity are present.

2. If such a youngster is a boy, the chance is three or four times as great as for a girl.

3. Should this child belong to a family in which there are known dyslexics, and if despite intellectual competence he is late in identifying letters and in placing them the right way up, the likelihood that he is a "pre-dyslexic" is great.

4. If crossed laterality happens to be demonstrated as well, then the risk is higher still.

5. Should there be no positive family history of developmental dyslexia and the child not only fails to identify letters and to orientate them correctly in space, but also shows such features as clumsiness, fidgetiness, reduced span of attention, belated acquisition of spoken speech and late arrival at the developmental milestones, the diagnosis is likely to be an overall learning-disability due to minimal cerebral dysfunction. Developmental dyslexia is unlikely in these circumstances, and if reading retardation stands out as the most conspicuous feature, the diagnosis of a "secondary" or "symptomatic" dyslexia may perhaps be justified.

Chapter Six

Dyslexics are not necessarily clumsy

"Undoubtedly clumsy children can be helped to overcome their difficulties. The trouble is that there are so few remedial facilities, but the more often the problem is diagnosed, so the pressure to find remedies will increase. So there is hope—but it lies in the hands of parents to push: politely, politically, any way you like, but most of all, persistently".

Ian Jack. "Sunday Times" 17th November 1974

A dyslectic child is not as a rule clumsy, despite a common belief to the contrary. True, some parents may speak of their dyslectic child in this way, but a confusion of ideas may be the reason for doing so. Clumsiness in the technical sense refers to a lack of manual dexterity. What some parents probably mean when they refer to their child as clumsy, is a state of general *gaucherie* or awkwardness, which persons of any age may display irrespective of any difficulties with reading. Thus a young dyslexic may be criticized for bumping into furniture, letting things drop, breaking crockery, knocking over articles, and for messy table-habits. But phenomena of this sort are something apart from his dyslexia, a personality trait perhaps, and entirely coincidental.

The syndrome of the "clumsy child" is familiar to neurologists and paediatricians, but it is not a clean-cut entity. When Walton (1965) and his associates wrote on this subject, they confessed to difficulty in defining it. The term "clumsiness" refers not so much to a lack of wide-range co-ordination as to a defect in fine finger-skills, coupled with an inability to perform rapidly alternating movements elegantly. The syndrome was probably described first by S. T. Orton in 1937. Ford (1959) referred to children of good intelligence who nevertheless were unable to learn complex motor activities, calling it "congenital maladroitness". He suggested that such cases might represent a specific developmental defect. Gubbay *et al* (1965) correlated the motor defects in their series of clumsy children with manifestations of an agnosic or

89

apraxic character which were, in fact, psychomotor features of a congenital nature. In a later paper, Gubbay (1973) said that the clumsy child is one whose ability to perform skilled movement is impaired, despite adequate intelligence and bodily configuration, the patient being virtually normal according to any standard of routine, conventional, and neurological assessment. As an alternative, and presumably as an explanation, he suggested that one might speak of such children as showing a "developmental apraxia and agnosia". He carried out a survey of 1,000 children aged between 6 and 12 years living in Western Australia; a series of eight tests were used and 50 children were studied in detail. He found they had educational, neurological and electrophysiological features which distinguished them from their peers.

Clumsiness, in the strict sense of the word, can be tested with or without the manipulation of toys or other articles. One may watch the manner in which a child assembles units of Lego, builds bricks one on top of another, ties and unties a knot in a piece of string, or fits shapes into form-boards. Clumsiness may also be demonstrated by the use of crayons for colouring outline drawings, if the result is a scribble which does not keep within the confines of the printed model. A doctor also tests a child's dexterity by getting him to carry out rapidly alternating movements with his hands and fingers, that is, opening and shutting one hand after another, or tapping the arm of the chair in which he is seated. A manoeuvre which taxes his skill even more, is for him rapidly to place the thumb on each finger-tip of one hand in turn, starting with the little finger. The examiner first demonstrates what is required, and the patient follows with the right hand first. When directed to perform similar movements with the left hand, the child often makes a spontaneous modification by opposing the thumb first to the tip of the forefinger (instead of the fourth), and then proceeds to touch the second, then the third and finally the fourth finger-tips. Just why he should carry out this test one way with the right hand and then another way with the left is obscure. Older children usually copy the examiner accurately and put the thumb first to the tip of the little finger and thereafter the others in sequence.

It is noteworthy, too, that children in the age-group of six to eight years manipulate the master hand, which is usually the right, better. Most older children, however, perform this test as well with either hand.

Another sign of clumsiness, and incidentally of motor immaturity, is the phenomenon of imitative synkinesis. That is to say, when the young child makes a difficult or a forceful movement with one hand, the other hand may often be seen to be making an involuntary small-range mirror-movement. It is best seen in a vigorous action like a hand-grip. If the examiner's index and middle fingers are squeezed hard by the child's right hand, the fingers of the left hand can often be seen to flex slowly. It may, incidentally, be necessary to stop him bringing his left hand into supportive action so as to squeeze the examiner's fingers tighter.

"Synkinetic" flexion of one hand during the execution of a forceful grasping movement with the other, is something which a normal child outgrows by the age of eight or nine. There may be a brief stage, however, during which he will carry out a grasping movement with the right hand and at the same make a slow and unwilled movement of *opening* the other hand. This represents a non-imitative or "inverse synkinesia".

It is natural for some degree of manuo-digital awkwardness to be present in the very young, for skilled movements develop only as a child grows older. A knowledge of what happens in normal children is essential, but neuro-paediatricians admit that their scales of motor maturation are only approximate. Children who are late in general development, however, continue to be maladroit in their small range movements longer than is usual.

If a case is said to belong to the category of the clumsy child, it is imperative to observe whether the lack of dexterity or faulty co-ordination waxes or wanes over a period of time. If it grows worse as the child gets older, the suspicion increases that some underlying neurological disorder might be present.

The conclusions arrived at by Gubbay and some others, are not convincing. To use the term "clumsy child" as a diagnosis is not entirely satisfactory, as it may represent merely a symptom of one of many neurological conditions such as progressive cerebellar ataxia—hereditary or otherwise; "congenital apraxia"; Louis-Bar's syndrome of ataxia telangiectasia; minimal diplegia; which is by no means an exhaustive list.

In those rare cases when a developmental dyslexic also shows true clumsiness, it is probably coincidental. Clumsiness is often included among those diverse attributes which have received in America the label of "soft" neurological signs, (to be described more fully in Chapter 11). When clumsiness or imperfect coordination constitute an enduring feature in a child with a learning-disability, one should strongly suspect that the dyslexia is a symptom of minimal brain-dysfunction and is not of the specific developmental variety.

When it comes to remedial therapy for developmental dyslexia, there is no logical place in the curriculum for elaborate systems of motor training. Physical exercises serve no greater role in the education of a poor reader than a welcome interlude to break up the tedium of overlong concentration upon difficult and demanding intellectual tasks. Even in the case of the late learner who is brain-damaged, physical exercises do not assist him with learning to read or with any other scholastic difficulties, however useful they may be in fostering motor-skills.

Both reading and the process of learning to read and write are functions of the whole brain: motor-skills are controlled by a relatively limited area. It is not reasonable to believe that learning to read or write can be facilitated by active movements of the limbs, or for that matter of the muscles of the eyes.

As stated earlier, clumsiness in developmental dyslexics is not only coincidental, but rare. A great many dyslectic boys are adept at model-making and at mechanical pursuits, and this expertise cannot be regarded as merely a projection or unconscious channelling of their interests away from books. Dyslectic boys often excel at ball-games. Dyslectic girls may be particularly proficient at sewing and needlework; some are pupil ballet dancers of promise. Given the opportunity, most boys and girls with developmental dyslexia are competent at riding and at swimming. The majority learn to ride a bicycle with great rapidity. Many dyslexics, though certainly not all, are above average in their ability to draw and to paint, and not a few in later life have become commercial artists or draughtsmen.

If clumsiness is such a rare concomitant of developmental dyslexia, why—it may be asked—are so many victims slovenly writers?

It is the exception rather than the rule for a dyslexic to write with impressive neatness. However, one must not assume that illegible or atrocious handwriting is necessarily an index of clumsiness. Not every brain-surgeon or ophthalmologist, however deft, is endowed with tidy or even readable handwriting. The untidy writing which is characteristic of so many children with developmental dyslexia, and incidentally many non-dyslexics too, often passes without undue comment from teachers. A generation or two ago, great attention was paid to the art of penmanship, but it seems now that a certain latitude exists in this field. As a dyslexic grows older he is likely to find that his untidy writing adds to his overall poor performance on paper. During the examination

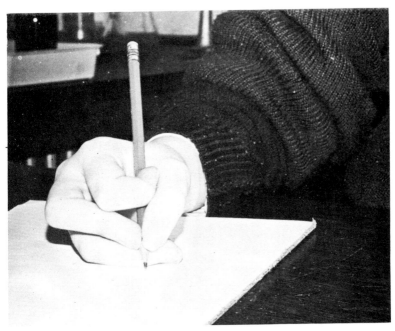

Fig. 23 Awkward hand-posture adopted while writing.

of such a patient, a note should be made whether the pen is held in an unorthodox fashion. Correction of this fault might obviate at least one of a dyslexic's handicaps. Instruction in the manipulation of a pen is a far more rational procedure than the use of bodily exercises as a means of overcoming alleged clumsiness or incoordination of the hands, for the mechanical act of handwriting is essentially a motor-skill affecting posture as well as coordination of upper limb and finger-movements; but it must be remembered that the basic problem is a cognitive one, transcending faulty pencil-grip or inadequate teaching of penmanship.

Chapter Seven

Cerebral dominance in dyslexics: is "crossed laterality" significant?

"*Sir, it is no matter what you teach them first, any more than what leg you shall put into your breeches first*".

Samuel Johnson

"*Many, in their infancy, are sinistrously disposed, and divers continue all their lives left-handed*".

Sir Thomas Browne

"*A wise man's understanding is at his right hand, but a fool's heart is at his left*".

Eccl. X, 2

It is not unknown for the parents of a dyslectic child to receive a written report couched in terms something like this:

"*. . because of his slight visual disability your little boy is left-handed but right-eyed and this makes him crossed lateral. The predicament of the crossed lateral child seems to lie in an inner conflict between sensory perception and motor activity in respect of the left-right rule of printed English. Some children find it extremely difficult to comprehend the pattern presented to them by the printed word and Jimmy is unable to perceive word patterns long enough for him to reproduce them when required. Often a child's crossed laterality leads to clumsiness, particularly in games where quick directional decisions must be made. It is invaluable for such children to learn to swim, to ride a bicycle and to try to play a musical instrument. All these are bilateral activities and develop bodily coordination.*"

These few sentences express certain ideas which, when not muddled, are untenable.

The myth of crossed laterality as something detrimental to the learning process, needs to be dispelled. Sometimes the term is used as though it were a concrete entity, and that in itself it is harmful and needs to be corrected. Parents often say "My child is crossed lateral", believing that the label is a medical diagnosis.

94

The idea is perpetuated by the existence of "Crossed laterality Clinics". It does not make sense. The sheer improbability that crossed laterality is a pathological condition is shown by the observation that it appears in the normal population in the ratio of approximately 3:7 (M. A. Clark 1957). Discounting any possible differences between right- and left-handers, Subirana had previously found in a group of 316 children, a "lack of concordance" (i.e. crossed laterality) in 143, or 45 per cent. (1952). But in order to dismiss the bogey that crossed laterality is abnormal, some discussion and explanation are required.

First, what is crossed laterality? It is a term employed to denote the product of a lack of firm superiority of one half of the brain over the other, although the underlying physiological mechanisms are obscure even to scientists who have studied the subject deeply. A child who holds his pencil in the right hand and also uses his right hand for automatic and unplanned actions like throwing a ball or chasing away an irritating fly, is in all probability right handed. Furthermore, if he chooses the right foot rather than the left to remove an obstacle from his path, or to take a penalty kick on the football field, he can fairly be judged to be right footed. Ordinarily we expect right handed persons to be right footed as well. Hopping is not a good test, because most children elect to hop on the left foot even when they are not left-footed. When it comes to one-sided visual activities like using a microscope or a telescope, or peering through a keyhole, it is natural to use one eye rather than the other. Most subjects who are right handed and right footed will, in such circumstances, employ the right eye.

Normally, then, a natural bond exists between the three preferences concerning handedness, footedness, and eyedness. Should the person belong to that minority group of natural sinistrals, then one would reasonably expect that not only would the left hand and the left foot be used in preference to the right, but that in all one-eyed procedures he would automatically employ the left eye.

If, however, the right handed, right footed child should happen to use the left eye rather than the right, he would be regarded as a crossed lateral. And yet, until specifically tested, the subject is usually unaware that one eye is the "ruling" eye, and the demonstration that he is a crossed lateral may in these circumstances come as a surprise both to the child and to his parents.

So far everything is straightforward, but there are certain underlying difficulties. Take, for example, the decision as to which is the ruling or master eye. It might be argued that an individual is left eyed because he has a relative defect of vision that involves the other eye: the "good" eye would, therefore, become the one which takes precedence. This is a serious objection and, if sustained, would go far towards invalidating the notion of a natural eye-preference, and thereby the whole concept of crossed laterality. However, ophthalmological experience has shown that minor degrees of poor vision in one eye do not necessarily imply that the better eye is the one chosen for uniocular activities. With more severe visual defects in one eye, matters may, however, be quite different.

Another complicating factor is less obvious. Usually, though not always, a scientist working with a telescope or a microscope uses one eye and closes the other. This practice, however, is not universal, for a student is sometimes instructed to keep both eyes open while using a microscope. Or, he might wish to take notes or sketches of what he is viewing, and, therefore, uses a pencil in his right hand while peering with the left eye. There is yet another complication. When specifically tested, some persons find it difficult to close one eyelid alone. Many can wink the right eye but not the left; or perhaps they can wink with either eye but do so more easily with the right rather than left; or it may be the other way round. The question then arises whether a person is left-eyed by reason of the fact that he can close only the right eyelid, or because the right eyelid can be closed more easily than the left.

This hypothesis deserves to be explored, but the series of test-subjects must be large enough for the results to be statistically significant. From our total series, a random selection of 248 children was made. All were poor readers and confirmed as cases of developmental dyslexia. The findings on their eyedness and ability to wink are set out below:

TABLE I

	Total	Boys 192	Girls 56
Could wink Right eye only	20	17	3
dominant eye right		6	1
dominant eye left		11	2
crossed lateral	11	8	3
not crossed lateral	9	9	—

Table I (continued)	Total	Boys 192	Girls 56
Could wink Left eye only	36	27	9
dominant eye right		24	9
dominant eye left		3	–
crossed lateral	11	10	1
not crossed lateral	17	9	8
Winking Right > Left	75	59	16
dominant eye right	41	31	10
dominant eye left		28	6
crossed lateral	28	24	4
not crossed lateral	47	35	12
Winking Left > Right	63	50	13
dominant eye right		35	12
dominant eye left		15	1
crossed lateral	15	14	1
not crossed lateral	48	36	12
Winking Right > Left	39	30	9
dominant eye right		25	7
dominant eye left		5	2
crossed lateral	5	3	2
not crossed lateral	34	27	7
Could not wink with either eye	15	9	6
dominant eye right		4	2
dominant eye left		5	4
crossed lateral	8	4	4
not crossed lateral	7	5	2

Thus of the total series of 248 children, 93 or 37·5 per cent were crossed laterals (boys 40·6 per cent; girls 26·7 per cent). These figures are higher than in the case of a non-dyslectic community.

It appears conceivable, therefore, that eyelid-closure may play some part in determining which eye is chosen for uniocular activities. Thus in 153 subjects who could either close one eyelid only, or else could close one more easily than the other, the preferred eye was the opposite one to the preferred eyelid in 98 examples, as opposed to 55 cases when the master eye was on the same side as the "master eyelid".

Nothing, incidentally, is known as to why one eyelid alone can be closed, or even why one eyelid should be easier to close than the other. These facts come to light only on specific testing. The ability or non-ability to wink is perhaps just one of the idiosyncratic facial phenomena that we cannot explain, like being able voluntarily to move the ears, or to elevate one eyebrow alone. It probably has nothing to do with cerebral dominance.

So much for ocular preferences: what about other types of incongruity? A person may be right handed and right eyed, but nonetheless prefers to kick with his left foot. Is he a crossed lateral? In theory he is, although the term crossed laterality implies that it is the eye which is the organ that does not conform to one-sided preference.

It now becomes necessary to explain what is meant by "cerebral dominance".

Man's brain, like that of most mammals, is a bi-lobed structure, a double organ. We know that each half controls voluntary or willed movements of the opposite side of the body, or, more accurately, of the contralateral limbs and lower part of the face. It also receives and stores sensory messages from that half of the body. Furthermore, each hemisphere is concerned with half-vision, that is, the outer half of the opposite side, and the inner aspect of the visual field on the same side. This crossed functioning of the brain applies to all mammals, including man, and also some submammalian creatures.

The conception of cerebral "dominance" began with the evolution of man. Both halves of the brain are alike with regard to the control of motor activity, sensory and visual perception. but a functional difference exists between the two sides of man's brain, the left hemisphere being particularly concerned with the faculty of language. For this reason one speaks of the left as the dominant hemisphere when dealing with right-handers, who, of course, make up the majority of the population. In the case of a truly left-handed person, it is presumed that the right half of the brain constitutes the dominant hemisphere.

At birth an infant does not show any manual predilection; that is, no unileral cerebral dominance exists. But after a few months he begins to display a tendency to move one limb more readily than the other, and later grasps objects more often in one hand. Parents may soon play a complicating role by encouraging the child to use one hand in particular. Most children grow up to be recognisable and established right-handers.

However, the two sides of the infant's brain mature at different rates. By the time the child is about 12 years of age, one half of the brain, usually the left, has become more concerned than the other with the function of language. In other words, it is attaining more significance and is taking on a greater load in some important respects. For this reason the left side of the brain is spoken of as constituting the dominant hemisphere in a right hander. By now a correlation has grown up between right handedness, the power of speech and the dominance of the left cerebral hemisphere. Can it be said which is responsible for what? Is the superiority of the left half of the brain the factor which determines the child's handedness? Or is it because he is right handed that the corresponding and controlling left hemisphere achieves greater importance than the right, with special reference to speech? These are fundamental questions which even now we cannot answer with confidence.

In what way does this concern the late reader?

In 1925 Samuel T. Orton emphasized that not all dyslexics are firmly right handed. Some are left handers—more, in fact, than would be expected in the general population; others have an ambiguous or indeterminate handedness. These facts, coupled with the notorious tendency of all dyslexics to be unduly late in discriminating between right and left, and quite often to rotate letters when writing, to reverse words, and perhaps even to perpetrate mirror-writing, led Orton to interesting though speculative ideas. He believed that the mechanism responsible for these tendencies lay in a delay in the attainment of precedence by one occipital lobe of the brain over the other, a phenomenon which ordinarily occurs in babyhood. In other words, he said, an equipotentiality of the two hemispheres continues for an unduly long period of time.

Subsequent work has confirmed Orton's ideas but without his hypotheses being accepted *in toto*, though the evidence is largely built up on impressions rather than statistics. Few workers have had an opportunity to test a large enough series of dyslexics, and afterwards correlating their findings with those obtained from a control series of non-dyslectic children of comparable age.

The figures complied by C. Burt (1946, 2nd Edition) showed that in his series of school-children who were left-handed, there was a sex-difference. Of his five thousand youngsters, he found that 5·8 per cent of boys and 3·7 per cent of girls were left-handed, as judged by the way they used a pencil. There was another difference, which was associated with intelligence. Out of the group of "backward" children, 9·6 per cent of boys and 6 per cent of girls were left-handed, while in the group of "educationally subnormal" children, the incidence of sinistrality was as high as 13·5 per cent among boys and 10·3 per cent among girls.

Another important analysis of "normal" children was carried out by Dr. Margaret Clark in 1957. In her series of 4,016 Scottish youngsters aged between ten and eleven years, 5·5 per cent were left handed. There was a minor sex difference, for of the 2,434 boys, 6·68 per cent were left handed, and of 1,582 girls, 4·41 per cent. The figures were then broken down according to regional and socio-educational factors. The percentage of left-handers in a community that lived in sparsely populated heath and moorland areas was as low as 4·76. However, the incidence of left-handedness was no less than 7·87 per cent among children attending private schools in Scotland. This discrepancy is difficult to explain. Moreover, no reference was made to the reading ability of the children surveyed.

Unfortunately many compilers have not explained their criteria when they used the terms right and left handedness. This raises a very important question, one which is particularly relevant to the observations made by S. T. Orton. Just what constitutes the evidence for handedness in a child or adult?

It has been said, and with justification, that there is no single test which proves beyond all doubt whether a person is right- or left-handed. A considerable battery of different techniques is needed to determine a subject's probable handedness.

The most usual index of laterality is taken as the hand which is chosen for writing. This is an important isolated indication, but it is not conclusive. Many a left-handed child has been forced to write and draw with the right hand even though all his instincts were to wield the pencil with the left hand. The practice of switching hands and producing a "shifted sinistral" is fortunately becoming rarer, but it has not yet entirely disappeared. Consequently it would be rash to assume that every person who writes or draws with the right hand is a "natural" right hander.

Some bimanual activities entail a different posture and pattern of behaviour in the two participating hands. It is conventional to distinguish a right-handed from a left-handed manner of performing skills such as using a spade or shovel. At cricket or baseball there is a characteristic stance. Even this cannot be taken as a wholly reliable testimony of innate handedness, for the natural left-hander might have been deliberately encouraged to play in an orthodox fashion. Boxing may be different. A sinistral tends to adopt a southpaw attitude, with the right arm and shoulder advanced, and when this technique is used naturally, it is usually encouraged. In dealing cards, a player holds the pack with one hand and distributes the card with the other. Like the stance of a boxer, it is probably an automatic action independent of prior instruction. Most right handers hold the pack in the left hand and deal with the right, but there are many exceptions, for quite a few strongly right handed persons deal cards in a sinistral manner. According to Freud, this denotes an unconscious desire to cheat.

Some acquired skills are fallible indicators of handedness for another reason. Racio-religious taboos may complicate the picture and the left is denigrated as the "wrong", the sinister, or the unclean hand. While the left hand may be used for purposes of personal toilet, it must never participate in feeding. This applies whether the subject eats with his fingers or with an implement. The same superstition applies to chopsticks. No Chinese, however naturally left handed, would ever use chopsticks except with the right hand.

A number of automatic actions or postures may possibly be correlated with handedness. These include the manner of folding one's arms; of clasping the hands together with fingers interlaced; of placing the hands behind the back when standing erect; and of clapping hands as when applauding.

Arm-folding is a difficult manoeuvre for a child below the age of 6½ years. After that, the so-called right handed manner of folding the arms is to tuck the master hand into one armpit, and to leave the non-dominant hand exposed.

When clasping the two hands with the fingers interlaced, the strongly right handed subject usually places the thumb of the non-dominant hand above the other thumb, that the little finger of the master hand occupies the lowermost position.

In standing with hands held behind the back, a right handed person ordinarily places the master hand on his left.

It is likely that the act of hand-clapping is carried out asymmetrically, that is, with one hand doing more work than the other. Insufficient information is available as yet to be confident that this is a useful test of handedness.

Automatic two-handed actions are easy to observe and require no tools or apparatus. Unfortunately there is no correlation with the writing hand, as shown in the following table:

Out of *151 right handed girls* who were tested and who use the right hand for writing:

   33 were "congruous" in that they also folded their arms and clasped their hands in a so-called right handed way. However,

 118 were "incongruous" in that they showed various types of inconsistency, viz:

   36 wrote with right hand, but folded arms left and clasped left:

   45 wrote with right hand, folded arms right and clasped hands left: and

   37 wrote with right hand, folded arms left, and clasped hands left.

Of *401 boys who used their right hands* for writing:

 112 were "congruous" in that they also folded their arms and clasped their hands in an allegedly right handed way.

 289 however, were "incongruous" for

   80 wrote with right hand, folded arms left and clasped hands left:

   56 wrote with right hand, folded arms right, and clasped hands left: and

 153 wrote with right hand, folded arms left, and clasped hands right.

Combining the figures for boys and girls, out of the *552 children who wrote with the right hand:*

 145 wrote, folded arms, and clasped hands in a consistently right handed manner, but

 407 were "incongruous". Of this latter number,

 116 wrote with right hand, folded arms and clasped hands in a left handed manner:

 101 wrote with right hand, folded arms in a right handed style, and clasped their hands left: while

189 wrote with right hand, folded arms left, and clasped hands right.

It appears as though a triple pattern of handedness is the exception, *concordance occurring in only 27 per cent.*

If one combines *two* of these items it will be seen that boys with a preferred right writing hand and right clasp make up 66 per cent of the cases, but in girls only 45 per cent. A combination of right handedness for writing and a right handed manner of folding arms occurred in 41 per cent boys and 51 per cent girls.

What about those *children who prefer to use their left hand for writing?*

Out of *92* such boys, 25 were "congruous" in that they wrote with the left hand, folded their arms in a left handed manner, and clasped their hands in a left handed fashion. It follows that 67 were "incongruous":

16 wrote with the left, folded arms right,
    clasped hands left.

24 wrote with the left, folded arms left,
    clasped hands right.

27 wrote with the left, folded arms right,
    clasped hands right.

Out of *32* girls who wrote with the left hand, 10 were "congruous" in that they wrote, folded arms and clasped hands in a left handed fashion. This means that 22 were "incongruous." Thus:

1 wrote with the left, folded arms right,
    clasped hands left.

7 wrote with the left, folded arms left,
    clasped hands right.

14 wrote with the left, folded arms right,
    clasped hands right.

Combining the figures for boys and girls who wrote with the left hand, of 124 such children 35 were "congruous" and 89 "incongruous", as follows:

17 wrote with the left, folded arms right,
    clasped hands left.

31 wrote with the left, folded arms left,
    clasped hands right.

41 wrote with the left, folded arms right,
    clasped hands right.

Again, taking two items rather than three, writing hand and hand-clasp went together in 17 or 53 per cent and writing hand

and arm-folding in 11 or 34 per cent. In boys, writing hand and clasping hand were the same in 41 instances, or 44 per cent; and writing hand and arm-folding in 48, or 52 per cent.

It appears, therefore, that neither the manner of folding arms nor of clasping the hands alone can be accepted as a reliable index of handedness.

It should be borne in mind that each of the 552 children tested had reading-problems, nearly all of them being true cases of developmental dyslexia. This fact may account for the surprisingly high incidence of left-handedness, i.e. 22·4 per cent.

Statistical significance might possibly emerge by correlating the writing hand with the manner of hand-holding behind the back, or of clapping hands. These possibilities have not yet been studied.

Perhaps the most reliable single test of hand-preference is to be found in the manner in which a nail-brush is employed. A genuine right-hander scours the nails of the left hand with the brush in his right hand. However, he holds the nail-brush immobile in the left hand, and cleans the nails of the other hand by moving the right hand rapidly up and down. A true left-hander behaves in the opposite manner. Most children of 6½ or less find the manoeuvre of nail-brushing unnatural and difficult. They often go through a phase of awkwardly moving both hands alternately up and down. By the age of seven, however, most of the difficulties have been resolved and the asymmetrical technique described above has been adopted and maintained throughout life.

There are rare exceptions and occasionally a child otherwise regarded as right handed, brushes his nails in an ambidextrous fashion. When this is so, it often transpires that there is a strong family history of sinistrality. In such subjects, left-handedness represents what Foster Kennedy described as "stock brainedness".

Some writers have said that it is possible to determine a child's master hand without relying upon which hand is used for writing (which, as already stated, might be artificially induced) or for any other motor-skill. They depend upon a relative diminution in the "tonus" of the muscles of the non-preferred limb. This can be demonstrated by passively moving the various joints of the two upper limbs. Diminished tonus is displayed by passively bending the subject's elbow-joint as far as possible, so that the forearm and upper arm take up a more acute angle. Or the child's thumb may be pushed back; it will be found that on one side it can be moved into an acute angle with the forearm. Ordinarily the more acute angles are obtained on the side which is not the preferred one, and where the muscle-tone is less.

A more simple test is to ask the child to make rapid finger movements first with one hand, and then with the other. The easiest manoeuvre is for him to place the tip of the thumb as rapidly as possible on the tip of each finger in turn. A difference in speed and agility on the two sides is often evident, the preferred or master hand being more dextrous than the other. Such a difference is less distinct in adults, especially if they have acquired bimanual skills such as typing, or playing the violin or piano.

Eventually we may no longer speak of right-handers and left-handers. Instead, we will be able to measure *degrees* of right or left preference. In technical jargon, handedness is not discrete or dichotomous, but a continuous variable. A person might turn out to be, say, 75 per cent right-handed and 25 per cent left-handed; or it might be 15 per cent right-handed and 85 per cent left-handed. In the latter event, we would probably look upon the subject as being a sinistral. This conception of degrees of handedness, which is steadily growing in acceptance, makes it difficult to estimate with confidence the percentage of sinistrals (or of crossed laterals) within any community.

The most recent and the most authoritative work on this subject has been by Subirana (1969). Realising the importance of a battery of tests in deciding manual preference, he estimated that pure and absolute right-handers make up about one quarter of the population. A pure left-handed person is extremely rare, and such a condition, he said, must always be suspected as being of pathological origin. But almost one in ten of the population who are allegedly left-handed subjects, nevertheless perform some of the tests with the right hand. The remainder have ambiguous preferences. Thus of a series of 271 subjects tested in detail, 38·7 per cent had a strong right-handed propensity and would be regarded by most authors as pure dextrads, while about one quarter (26·9 per cent) had "accentuated mixed preferences". Out of the whole series tested by Subirana, therefore, 2/3rds are purely or predominately right-handed, and one in ten is principally left-handed.

Of even greater interest and possible significance, in theory at any rate, is the direction of automatic gaze—a subject which was briefly touched upon by Orton. When one looks into the distance and examines or counts a series of objects on the horizon, one either looks first at the right extremity and then shifts the gaze to the left; or one can start at the left and deviate the gaze from left to right. Most adults as well as children, dyslexics and non-dyslexics, right-handers or sinistrals, automatically move their eyes from left to right in these circumstances. Could there possibly be some significance here? That is, do we automatically scan the horizon from left to right because we read that way? Or do we read in that fashion because our automatic gaze sweeps from left to right? We do not know. It would be of great interest to determine whether the same direction of automatic gaze also applies to literate members of those races which write in a sinistral fashion, e.g. Arabs, Israelis and Iranians. Such information is not yet available, and a potentially important research project stands ready. So far the amount of relevant information is scanty, but currently a routine testing of the direction of lateral gaze is being carried out on all individuals encountered whose mother-tongue is Arabic, Farsi, or Hebrew. The subjects tested have been of all ages, and mostly literate. To date the results are as follows:

	Automatic gaze	
	R. to L.	L. to R.
Arabs	47	44
Iranians	15	44
Israelis	1	1

Obviously these figures are too few, but, as far as they go, they show a somewhat greater proportion of right to left eye-movements in Arabs (mostly Iraquis) than is seen in English-speaking subjects.

Against the hypothesis that one's automatic gaze depends upon the direction of printed or written script, is the fact that automatic eye-movement from left to right is demonstrable in English children before they have learned to read. The same hypothesis of correlation between gaze and direction of language cannot apply to Chinese, where the print flows from above downwards, and from right to left. Ancient Assyrian, too, is read from above down, but from left to right. In the earliest Greek and Latin texts the writing, judged by inscriptions on stone, proceeded in a "plough-wise" fashion, that is, from left to right and from right to left in alternate lines. This is the so-called "boustrophedon" script, which only later settled down and became consistently dextrad in direction.

It is conceivable that those children whose gaze travels from right to left might find unusual difficulty in overcoming their confusion in right-left orientation, and in their tendency towards mirror reversals of letters and words. So far, however, there is no real evidence to support this speculative idea. Right-left automatic gaze is rare in England, and it does not seem to be associated closely with difficulties in reading.

So far, it has become obvious that some tests of laterality are more valuable than others, just as some tests of handedness are more valid than others. The time may well come when it will be feasible to evaluate by a precise "mark" each individual motor or ocular test. Furthermore, it might be possible to assess a "dominance quotient", whereby one could estimate each individual's *degree* of handedness, eyedness, and footedness. By taking into account comparable degrees of eye- and foot-preference, it should eventually be possible to evolve a formula which indicates the "dominance quotient", which might also turn out to show, say, 56 per cent left-brained as against 44 per cent right-brained superiority. From the results of multiple tests for handedness and so on over the course of years in individual dyslexics in our series, it appears probable that longitudinal studies may show a slight trend towards an increasing left-brained superiority. This conforms with present beliefs that left-handedness, and especially unstable laterality represents a state of relative immaturity from which the growing adolescent gradually emerges.

The concept of laterality may entail something more than a preference for one arm, one leg and one eye, for the sense of hearing may also be important (Bakker *et al*, 1973). It may be that one ear takes precedence over the other in picking up sounds and interpreting them. The idea is an attractive but a complicated one. At a cocktail party it is a common experience to be assailed by a volume of talk which impinges on the ears from in front, from behind, from the right and from the left. With luck one may be able to give most attention to one's neighbour although competing sounds bombard the ears from all sides. It is possible, indeed probable, that some outside items of conversation rather than others are picked up and serve as mental distractions. Perhaps the question of sidedness plays a part, and words and phrases heard in the left ear are a greater competition to one's efforts to concentrate than similar sounds coming from the right. If so, this might be looked upon as evidence of a left-ear preference; or it may be the other way round. This latter condition, we believe, normally applies to linguistic stimuli as opposed to non-linguistic noises.

More basic facts need to be established before any theory of ear-laterality can be established. First, is the acuity of hearing the same on the two sides? Although a person may believe that it is, precise audiometric testing may bring to light an impairment for high-tone sounds in one ear rather than the other. He may have been previously unaware of this fact, which might well make him more attentive to sounds impinging on the better side.

Secondly it is necessary to consider the type of sounds concerned. The mere decibel content, i.e. the simple factor of loudness, may be important, and sounds of great volume may take precedence over sounds which are more subdued. Another potentially important factor concerns pitch. The high-tone voices of women engaged in conversation may swamp the lower tones emanating from a group of men on the other side of the room.

Nowadays some of these variables can be analysed scientifically by means of the technique of "dichotic" listening. The subject wears headphones and sounds are played into each earpiece differing in loudness, pitch and quality. It is also possible to test whether speech fed into one earpiece competes with the opposite earphone into which various non-verbal sounds (hissing, ringing, clapping, whirring) may be played, or—most significant of all— music. The results are interesting and striking. Music played into one ear may "extinguish" words played into the other; or, conversely, human speech in one ear may direct attention away from melodies played into the opposite ear. Most workers in this field claim that the right ear is better at picking up speech, while the left is more sensitive to wordless music.

Interesting results have also been claimed when speech is used as a stimulus in both ears, that is, words which are different in content though comparable in pitch and loudness. It has been found that the right ear is quicker than the left in picking up the verbal stimuli, and also in identifying the words. The left ear is slower in these respects and also less accurate. As the right ear feeds information into the left half of the brain, that is, the one which is dominant for speech, the right ear may be looked upon as the "master ear" as far as language is concerned.

If these researches are confirmed, it means that the formula of "laterality dominance" will be even more complicated than originally supposed, and that in addition to degrees of handedness, footedness and eyedness, we must also take into account the element of earedness.

In "*The Dyslexic Child*" (1970) reference was made to the quest which has gone on over the years for some obvious anatomical clue to a person's cerebral dominance, which would make it possible, for example, to assert the life-time handedness of a corpse. So far nothing has been discovered short of dissection and accurate measurement of the skeleton. Reference was also made to an idea which had been put forward as a physical sign of laterality, namely the position of the hair-whorl. Ordinarily this lies a little to one side of the midline of the skull, and the suggestion was made that a left-sided hair-whorl correlates with right-handedness, and vice versa. This speculative notion was ingenious, but unfortunately does not accord with the facts. The hair-whorls of many hundreds of dyslectic children in our series were examined, but it has not been possible to demonstrate any association with handedness. Sometimes in fact it is not easy to determine exactly where the hair-whorl lies. Sometimes it is represented by a short horizontal oblique cleft; sometimes it is situated dead centre; and very occasionally there are two hair-whorls, one on either side of the midline. Or, in the case of the adult male, baldness may obliterate all previous traces of a hair-whorl.

An even more artless suggestion has been proffered, namely that the site of the hair-whorl is less important than the direction of the hairs emerging from it. It was hypothesized that a clockwise direction of the emerging hairs indicated right-handedness. This cannot be so because an anti-clockwise whorl must be rare indeed, and in our large-scale scrutiny not a single instance was seen.

It is worth mentioning that language-laterality, as opposed to handedness, can often be established by physiological procedures, some of them rather drastic. In the Wada test amylobarbitone is injected into a carotid artery, and a temporary loss of speech indicates which hemisphere is the dominant one. There is also the test of unilateral electroconvulsive shock (ECT), which indicates which side is concerned with speech. (Pratt and Warrington.) Fortunately the non-traumatic measure of dichotic listening, has lately been found to be potentially useful, as already described.

Some of these procedures sound Draconian, but they may be important when neurosurgical intervention is being planned. To date, however, they do not seem to have any significant bearing on the problem of reading.

How common is left-handedness within the general population? The figures in the literature range from one per cent to 30 per cent. Much depends upon whether by left-handedness one includes or disregards preferences as to the use of the eye and foot. Figures collected in the U.S.A. have shown that in a community of developing children, to every one who grows up to use the left hand by choice, 18 to 24 become confirmed right-handers. Differences are also found according to whether the index of left-handedness is the use of the hand for writing, or whether an elaborate battery of tests is employed. The work of Subirana, quoted earlier in this chapter, represents the most up-to-date opinion on this difficult topic.

At this point something should be said about the concept of ambidexterity. This is an expression sometimes used to indicate a lack of preference for either hand, manual skill being presumably equal on the two sides. Over the years increasing scepticism has grown up as to the very existence of such a state of affairs. Zangwill, for example, thought that such cases were really instances of "ambilevity", in that neither hand ever became completely deft, both always remaining a little maladroit. Earlier, Burt said that out of several cases of ambidexterity in children, only seven could be accepted, and furthermore that as a child grows older, ambidexterity proves to be almost non-existent.

As regards developmental dyslexia, most workers (though not all) find that the percentage of left-handers is relatively high. For example, in our sample group of 552 children with developmental dyslexia, 151 were deemed to be left-handed on the basis of their choice of that hand for writing. That is to say, 27 per cent were left-handed, and 73 per cent right-handed, figures which surely differ from the incidence in the general population. What is probably even more characteristic of dyslexics, is that many showed imperfect lateralisation with a larger battery of tests, one cerebral hemisphere failing to exercise a very firm dominance over the other. This was also the case in Harris' series (1957) where 40 per cent showed mixed dominance, and also in the Chesni series where the figure was 37 per cent.

In the Isle of Wight community studied by Rutter and his group (1975), there did not appear to be any correlation between sinistrality or ambiguous laterality and poor reading achievement. Eighty-six children between the ages of 9 and 11 fell into a category labelled "specific reading retardation". Mixed handedness was not found to be commoner among them than in the control population; the same applied to sinistrality. Rutter's cases, for this and other reasons which will be detailed in Chapter 12, are, unlikely to have been instances of specific developmental dyslexia.

Imperfect cerebral dominance includes crossed laterality, a condition which is probably commoner in dyslexics than in non-dyslexics. Unless the percentage of crossed laterals can be shown to be very high, it would be foolish to assert that either phenomenon is responsible for the other. It is more reasonable to think that the crossed laterality is nothing more than an epiphenomenon, and that both developmental dyslexia and crossed laterality stem from a common underlying factor, the most likely being a state of delayed and uneven cerebral maturation.

Without doubt a child may be a crossed lateral yet learn to read, write and spell at an early age and eventually attain considerable facility in the use of language. Crossed laterality is not the cause of imperfect reading, and, to return to the opening paragraphs in this chapter, it is not responsible for right-left disorientation. It does not give rise to clumsiness, which, as emphasized in Chapter 6, is relatively rare in children with specific developmental dyslexia. There is no need to urge the child to swim or bicycle as a remedial measure. The vast majority in our series of dyslexics swim well, and have learned to ride a bicycle with rapidity. When the opportunity arises, they also show skill at skiing and riding.

To burden a dyslexic with the additional task of learning to play a musical instrument on account of crossed laterality (as has been advocated in one paper) is unwise, for there is a risk of failure— not because of any bimanual incoordination but through the sheer inability of the child to sightread easily a musical score.

Many more questions arise in any discussion of handedness. It could be debated whether a right manual preference in *homo sapiens* is a phenomenon which is innate and built into the human nervous organism, or whether it is a belated faculty which develops naturally, or whether it is something that is acquired and hence the product of environmental circumstances. No definite answer is yet forthcoming, and it is not germane to the topic of developmental dyslexia to pursue this fascinating question further now.

Under the arresting title of "The advantages of being dyslexic", a theme has been ably and eloquently propounded by Masland (1975). He stressed the differences in function which are believed to exist between the dominant and the subordinate halves of the brain. He said there is good reason to believe that the minor hemisphere is more concerned with certain concepts and faculties than the major one, so that the non-dominant hemisphere is not just a feeble reflection of its fellow. Though the left half of the brain (in the right-handed majority) is particularly concerned with the faculty of language, the opposite side is more bound up with superior spatial notions and with non-linguistic perception, visual as well as auditory. Masland quoted Luria, who among others, regarded the right side of the brain as superior to the left for the analysis and coordination of sensory stimuli, so as to assist each one of us to orientate himself as well as surrounding objects in space. The left hemisphere is the one chiefly concerned with communication. If Orton was correct in believing that reading-retardation is the product of inadequate dominance of the left over the right half of the brain, then the dyslexic might well prove to be endowed with compensatory abilities of a mechanical rather than a linguistic sort. In other words, there may be subtle advantages in being dyslexic. To say this does not imply that when a dyslectic student slowly attains mastery over written words he loses the compensatory non-linguistic skills. Nor should it be used as an argument for withholding remedial teaching from a dyslexic.

Chapter Eight

Problems of the Ex-dyslexic

"We simply do not know much about the long-term effects of this handicap upon the lives of individuals. The extent to which the disorder persists into adulthood has not been consistently documented. Factors involved in the disappearance or continuation of a childhood reading disability are largely unknown".

B. M. Herjanic and E. C. Penick, 1972

"Given average or better intelligence, physical normality and equivalent social and educational opportunity in both groups, differences in educational and vocational achievement by adulthood on the part of non-dyslectic boys and dyslectic boys between the ages of six and twelve will not be greater than could be explained by chance alone".

M. B. Rawson, 1968

"I am word-blind. I can't read and I can't write. I get a headache and then I can't think. In school I was the worst in the class. I was not lazy, but I just couldn't read. It was such a big handicap for me".

Paul Elvström. (World Champion Racing yachtsman; four times Olympic gold medallist; professional sail-maker.)

"Elvström speaks."

Almost every parent of a dyslectic child must have worried about the nature of his child's disability, and what to expect from him when looking ahead ten or twenty years. Two questions are commonly asked at the end of a diagnostic interview. The first is not difficult to answer, and when a parent enquires whether there exist mild as well as severe cases of developmental dyslexia, the reply is readily made. Individuals vary as to the severity of their dyslexia. In some the disability is relatively trivial and transitory; in others—fortunately not many—it is persistent and occasionally even intractable to treatment. Most however, fall somewhere between the two extremes. The second question is far less easy, and that is how dyslectic children can be expected to fare later in

113

their school life; what examinations they will be likely to pass; and what sort of career will be open to them.

The reply has to take into account many factors, some environmental, others innate; some being favourable and others less so. Before discussing in detail this complexity of factors, two important matters must be considered.

First, if we believe developmental dyslexia to be a localized maturational lag of the learning processes, we should also expect the disability to lessen as the patient grows older. This view brings comfort and relief, but to offset such a sanguine thought comes the realisation that throughout the years of schooling, much of the day to day teaching must have passed over the dyslexic's head. Consequently, the adolescent, though then able to read acceptably well, will still be encumbered by a backlog of basic ignorance.

It is remarkable that despite the large number of dyslectic children who have been assessed, recorded, and treated, there is little precise information concerning prognosis. Since 1959 there have been fewer than a dozen known attempts at a follow-up study of a series of dyslexics over 10 to 20 years, in order to determine the outcome. The published results have not been impressive, for the divergencies in the sampling have been so wide. It is obvious that any long term study needs to embrace an unwieldy number of variables including personal and environmental factors as well as intellectual and socio-economic elements. In addition, the type, quality and duration of remediation must be considered. To embark adequately upon such a research-project requires a considerable population of fully assessed dyslexics and a comparable control-group. Detailed documentation as to management, care and remediation is necessary, and the resulting statistics would be complex. Such a study would need an adequate number of personnel, patients, and good facilities for recording data.

Encouragement can be derived from one particular follow-up study, namely that carried out in 1968 by Rawson. Admittedly the series was a highly selected one, but the results are so striking as to offer a promise of fulfilment which cannot be dismissed. Rawson's group was made up of 56 pupils (most of them, she said, being upper class) at an American private school, 20 of whom were moderately or severely dyslexic, and 16 mildly so. The boys continued at school for at least three years. The median I.Q. of the 56 scholars was as high as 131; specialized instruction was provided when deemed advisable. Twenty-three years later, all but ten of the 56 were working in the upper two socio-economic classes. Seven were in Class III, one in Class IV and two in Class V on the Werner scale. All pursued training beyond high school. Except one, all attended college, and 48 of the 56 attained degrees. While many of the "low language facility" group continued to experience difficulties in reading and spelling, they managed to find ways of circumventing their handicap.

Despite the lack of statistical data, clinical experience clearly shows that the prognosis in developmental dyslexia is influenced by two sets of factors, some favourable, others not. Of these, the former is the weightier.

On page 15 a brief reference was made to that constellation of circumstances which may be looked upon as favourable for the progress of the growing dyslexic. This "prognostic pentagon", is made up of five favourable factors, each of which is highly important and in conjunction are invaluable. They are the following:

(1) *The fundamental intellectual level.*
Ceteris paribus, it is undoubtedly an advantage for a dyslexic to be endowed with a superior intelligence quotient.

(2) *Early diagnosis.* The sooner accurate assessment is made, the better. Any emotional problems that happen also to be present must be evaluated, and a clear distinction arrived at between stresses that are secondary (that is, reactionary) and those which are primary or causative. The suspicion that structural brain-damage is present must also be allayed. Schoolroom misdiagnoses and misinterpretations such as "laziness", "stupidity", "day-dreaming", "inattention", have to be rated at their proper level and probably rejected. So too the accusation of over-anxious interference on the part of the parents.

(3) *A sympathetic and understanding attitude on the part of both teachers and parents.* This climate of empathy goes far to facilitate the upward progress of the dyslectic schoolchild. Such cooperation is not always encountered, for sometimes one comes across teachers who proclaim that they "do not believe in dyslexia"; that the boy is a "late developer" and "all will come right in the end". Occasionally, too, the father—much more often than the mother—is not altogether sympathetic, and resents the child's failure to shine academically.

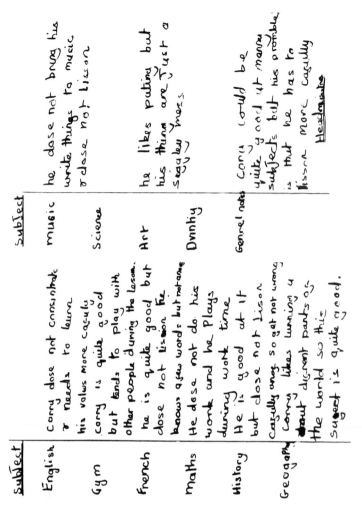

Fig. 24 An imaginary school report on a boy name Corry. Written by an atypical dyslectic girl aged 10.09 years (R.A. 12; Sp.A. — 10).

(4) *The availability and the institution of intensive, skilled, sympathetic tuition,* ideally on a one-to-one basis, by a teacher experienced in the modern techniques of remediation. Such assistance may not always be easy to find, but when help of this kind is available, the future is bright. Each lesson should be not too protracted, for learning to read is a more wearisome chore to a dyslexic than many

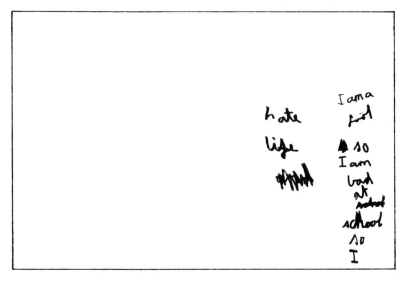

Fig. 25   Attitude of despair in a dyslectic boy of 10.05 years who had kept this letter partially concealed in his bedroom.

realise. Arnold Bennett had an inkling of this when he wrote "It is impossible to read properly without using all one's engine-power. If we are not tired after reading, commonsense is not with us". All important is a climate of warmth and understanding between teacher and pupil.

Many systems of remedial instruction are available, and some of them suit one patient better than another. Most teachers are broadminded and eclectic in their attitude, and the choice of approach may confidently be left to the experienced teacher.

(5) Lastly, and perhaps this is the most potent single factor, a *powerful drive towards attainment* is desirable. An ambition to master, by hook or by crook, the dull, tiring and baffling mystery of verbal symbols, is a vastly important personality-trait. It has been termed staying-power, ego-strength, or, more simply, "guts". Such an endowment probably enabled Hans Christian Andersen to conquer his near-illiteracy; and King Karl XI of Sweden to by-pass or cover up his problems with printed words.

The first and last of the foregoing factors, namely high intelligence and drive, probably explain the high achievement of those dyslexics in the past who had distressing difficulties with reading and writing in their youth and who despite the lack of skilled remediation as we know it today, achieved success.

To offset these propitious circumstances, there are a number of influences, some environmental, which are likely to retard a dyslexic's progress. It must be emphasized that these factors are not causal but merely unpropitious. They are diverse in nature and include others beside the converse of the five favourable factors.

Here we may mention three:—

(1) *A polyglot background.* When the parents are of different races and speak different languages there may be an attempt to bring up a child as a bilingual in the hope of him mastering both parental tongues with equal ease. Normally this practice would be acceptable. However, if the child is dyslexic the problem of coping equally well with two languages, that is, communication by audible speech and by the written word, will probably bring about unforeseen difficulties.

(2) *Inconsistent schooling.* This may be an unavoidable detriment, for some children change schools in rapid succession simply because their parents have to move from city to city or from one country to another. This happens in the case of diplomats, members of the armed forces, oil executives, and so on. It applies similarly to people engaged in the theatrical profession, to circus folk, to travelling showmen, and to gipsies.

(3) *Inadequate techniques of teaching* conceivably play a part. The nursery school-teacher who first introduces the child to its letters may happen to be inexperienced. Possibly unorthodox experimental techniques (such as i.t.a. or the look-say method) have been introduced. Among the more vocal critics of the concept of developmental dyslexia is Crabtree, who not only denies its existence but attributes all contemporary defects in literacy to faulty teaching-techniques, and in particular to the neglect of a phonic approach to reading.

The foregoing are merely examples. There are other personal or environmental circumstances which retard the educational progress of a dyslectic child, but most have already been mentioned in Chapter 2.

Initiating these remarks was the question of the eventual fate of a dyslectic child. This leads naturally to a rider: is a dyslexic ever cured?

A direct yes or no is not realistic, for the reply depends upon the criterion of the word "cure".

If "cure" implies the attainment of a standard of reading-ability which is acceptable within the community, then the answer is definitely yes. Experience over many years shows beyond all doubt that dyslexia need not debar a scholar from graduating at University, or from entering one of the learned professions, or thereafter achieving higher degrees and subsequent distinction.

Reservations there must be, however. To probe the linguistic life of the ex-dyslexic is to uncover a number of subtle flaws which may persist indefinitely. In the first place the ex-dyslexic, though able to read, may prefer not to, if there is an alternative. He may no longer be a reluctant reader, but, nonetheless he has joined the community of seldom readers. Apart from skimming through a newspaper, he rarely chooses to buy and avidly study a book. Outdoor pursuits; artistic or mechanico-technical work; administration; all may come easily to an ex-dyslexic. His leisure hours are occupied by doing things, rather than by reading. His personal stock of books is likely to be meagre. Rarely does he browse in secondhand bookshops or in reference libraries.

In the course of his profession he may find uncongenial the perusal of documents, reports, briefs, Parliamentary papers. If possible he will depute to his junior, his secretary, or his assistant, the task of providing him with a verbal summary. Lloyd George has been said to have shirked the task of wading through the multiplicity of papers, reports, and documents which confronted him, preferring to leave that duty to his team of secretaries who would digest them and retail the subject-matter to him. From various sources we have learned that he was a voracious reader, but always a slow one. He never attained mastery of French, and all his life he was an incorrigibly poor correspondent. Scores of unanswered letters would accumulate; many he never bothered to open and read. His old adversary, Georges Clemenceau, probably had an inkling of this, for he said "I am not sure whether Mr. Lloyd George *can* read, but I am sure he never does".

This is not to say that the ex-dyslexic may not amass a fairly rich word-bank, and not infrequently he is even endowed with the silver gift of tongues. Dyslexia does not debar the victim from achieving eminence as a conversationalist, an orator, preacher, lecturer or public speaker. In other words, he moves with facility within the confines of what we may call his "available" vocabulary. Ordinarily we possess two vocabularies, which are first the utilizable and secondly the utilized. The former refers to the storehouse of words which are not used very much but which are fully understood. They are only rarely employed in spoken speech, though more often in writing. This utilizable or available vocabulary is probably smaller in ex-dyslexics than in the case of the avid reader.

Some years ago a young adult dyslexic said her reading improved when she looked at the large print volumes published for the partially sighted. Mindful of the fact that the same phenomenon is encountered in some elderly patients who had lost their facility in reading after a stroke, a relatively easy text was typed in both lower case and upper case lettering. The two specimens were mounted on cards and presented to a series of our adolescent ex-dyslexics to read aloud. The results were not uniform. Some said that, within reasonable limits, the larger typefount made the task of identification easier. In view of the notorious difficulty experienced by most persons in hoisting in the meaning of the small print on policies, railway tickets and many other quasi-official leaflets, this finding caused no surprise. But some ex-dyslexics were in no doubt that the larger print was harder to read than the smaller version. They explained that as there were more words to a line when the typeface was small, the task of proceeding from word to word and particularly that of switching from the end of one line to the start of the next, was easier as well as less frequent in occurrence. There was a third group, where the patient did not find any real difference in comprehensibility between the small print and the large. As these categories were roughly equal in number, it was concluded that size of type was not an important factor in helping or hindering ex-dyslexics when reading.

The ex-dyslexic is liable to meet difficulties—and this is not unknown even in the case of non-dyslexic persons—in distinguishing certain words he has heard spoken or seen in print only rarely. Examples of pairs of words where the difference in meaning may be obscure to him include militate and mitigate; flaunt and flout; vicious circle and vicious cycle; resort and recourse.

The secret world of the ex-dyslexic contains yet another problem. He is probably an incorrigibly slow reader, and is unlikely to be helped by "rapid reading" courses. When the dyslectic individual reads aloud, a duty which he tends to shirk if possible, he is apt to stumble in the pronunciation of polysyllabic or unfamiliar terms. More often he puts the stress on the wrong syllable. In his limited reading the ex-dyslexic may have come across a particular word but has glossed over the stage of subvocal or silent articulation. Consequently he fails to correlate accurately the version as spoken by educated adults with the verbal symbol he has encountered in print and shied away from.

Thus in the diction of the ex-dyslexic (and, of course, in some ill-educated non-dyslexics), the accent often falls incorrectly on such words as dispute, formidable, voluntarily, controversy, research, coronary, lamentable; while frank errors occur with words like indictment, secretary, urine, vertigo, migraine, necessarily, opposite, and mischievous. Then there are such place-names as Woburn, Heysham, Frome, Congresbury, and many others.

The ex-dyslexic may blunder while reading aloud under stress. This sometimes occurs in the witness-box when the reluctant or seldom reader may falter in taking the Oath, or perusing documents or letters handed up to him and then having to read them aloud in Court. While at ease, however, he reads adequately.

When the ex-dyslexic tries to speed up his silent reading he is liable to make errors. Not only does he skip or misread relatively unfamiliar words but even the short "filler" terms—the articles, particles, prepositions and conjunctions. The consequence may be serious, especially if a negative statement is read as though it were an affirmation: a veritable travesty of comprehension may result. Ex-dyslexics recall the very real difficulty they probably encountered in making sense of the lengthy questions set out in their "O" and "A" level examination papers. These pitfalls are considered more fully in Chapter 10.

Such handicaps are by no means confined to the ex-dyslexic, for as emphasized in Chapter 3 all of us are potentially word-blind when confronted with a printed text that is unusually recondite or technical. Paragraphs of increasing complexity entail differing degrees of accurate legibility and comprehension.

The second hidden defect bedevilling an ex-dyslexic, betrays itself when he puts pen to paper. Not only is he a seldom reader, he is still more a timid writer. That is to say, he is an unsatisfactory correspondent: his letters are brief and often platitudinous. When writing reports or statements—the grim task of school essay-writing belonging now to the unhappy past—he still finds it far from easy to express his ideas on paper. It is a slow and irksome labour and the end-result lacks merit. Creative impulse may be forceful; he may be imaginative and original in his thinking, but the ideas are still-born when expressed on paper.

We have already stated that it is not impossible for an ex-dyslexic to become a public speaker of consummate eloquence. Even so, it is arguable that his harangues, if ever committed to print, would make disappointing reading. This should not be a matter for surprise, for the utilizable word-bank of the ex-dyslexic is likely to be relatively poor after years of attenuated reading.

The ex-dyslexic cannot always escape the duty of writing documents, but his speed is noticeably slow. During his schooldays and also at college, his ability to finish each answer in written examinations in the allotted time may have been a considerable handicap. In adult life, however, this may matter less.

The linguistic characteristics of the prose-writings of an ex-dyslexic have already been described (altered token-type ratio; anomalous verb-adjective fraction; low syllable-sentence count; etc.).

The shrewd ex-dyslexic will utilize manoeuvres like dictating to his secretary or into a tape-recorder. In such favourable circumstances, words tumble out and later and at his leisure they can be re-assembled and a preliminary draft made coherent.

Not many writers or poets are known to us who were obviously dyslexic during their schooldays. Hans Christian Andersen is a conspicuous exception, as is the journalist and script-writer Lord ("Ted") Willis, and the Danish novelist Sara Tomsen.

The third hallmark of the ex-dyslexic is inaccuracy in spelling, especially when he is tired. As in his schooldays the dyslexic is still uncertain how seldom used words should be spelt, and in his errors he betrays the same inconsistencies. Reversals are far less common in the writings of an ex-dyslexic. He may, however, still fail to recognise the mistake in a mis-spelt text when he looks at it. By now, the ex-dyslexic is well aware of his difficulties, and in writing letters he may realise that the word he wishes to use is one he cannot spell. He searches in his mind for a simpler alternative, and this mental exercise retards him even more.

Though now an adult, the ex-dyslexic will still not have wholly overcome his earlier difficulties with sequencing. The troubles are less blatant, however, and such serial concepts as the order of days of the week and months of the year have now become well established. He probably continues to find it rather a slow business to consult a dictionary or to look up a name in a telephone directory, and he avoids these tasks as far as possible. The ex-dyslexic might become worried when having to file records in alphabetical order, or to retrieve papers that have been already put away, and he may not be entirely successful in this task.

Eventually most dyslectic adults come to terms with their integral problems and accept them good humouredly or make adequate compensation. They will then have lost most of the frustration, the lack of self-confidence, the sense of inferiority or of bitterness which may have coloured their schooldays. They are able to take a detached view of their earlier difficulties, and by so doing are in a position to contribute much to our understanding of a dyslexic's dilemmas and their solution.

Finally, it should be said that the term "ex-dyslexic" might be liable to misinterpretation, and, therefore, is probably not an ideal expression. It is used when the early reading difficulties have been overcome although erratic spelling and slow poor writing persist. However, the residual difficulties are usually not severe enough for the label "dyslexic" to be used for life.

Chapter Nine

Dyslexia-equivalents: dyslexia variants

"Typical syndromes are usually either congenital, familial or hereditary and are the result of genetic abnormality. These variations depend upon the presence of a single pleiotrophic gene or of two or three linked genes. Not infrequently such inherited abnormalities include an inexplicable combination of two, three, or even four seemingly unrelated conditions . . . In some instances the manifestations of a syndrome are incomplete; this partial anomalism is known as formes frustes. *On occasion, a syndrome may occur within a syndrome . . ."*

Robert H. Durham (1960)

"It is not at all rare in psychological medicine that a disease should have no unique identifying sign, that uniqueness being in the pattern of signs that appear in contiguity. Out of context, each sign might be encountered in other diseases, or, in different intensities, in the healthy".

John Money (1962)

Children are often referred to a doctor on account of a learning-disorder or because of inadequacies in written work, where development dyslexia seems at first sight not to be the obvious diagnosis, if only because the individual's ability to read conforms with both chronological age and intelligence. Might it be that such cases, or at least some of them, can still be looked upon as falling within a rather broader conception of the syndrome of developmental dyslexia? In other words, can they be considered as dyslexia-variants? If so, they are certainly fewer in number than the classic instances of the syndrome.

The suspicion that certain unusual forms of linguistic retardation may in reality be *formes frustes* of developmental dyslexia, becomes all the greater when there are one or two members of the family who are indubitable cases.

Perhaps the most conspicuous of the possible variants of dyslexia is the "pure" or "specific" spelling-disability, as it is often called.

Melvin Cole (1964) used the expression "special educational disability involving spelling".

Not infrequently one finds a boy or girl whose written work is marred by erratic and inconsistent spelling. Some of the errors are so outlandish as to baffle interpretation of the text, and yet the parents insist that their child had not been late in learning to read, and that he reads well, rapidly and with enjoyment. Furthermore they say he can express himself in both written and spoken speech fluently and logically. These are the cases where some writers have visualised a developmental spelling-disability existing as an entity *sui generis*.

Another interesting experience when taking the history of a child with developmental dyslexia, is to find one parent—perhaps more often the mother—admitting that she has always been a highly unorthodox speller, even though a voracious and an early reader.

Are such allegedly "pure" cases of spelling-disability in fact variants of developmental dyslexia? The evidence is suggestive enough to raise the suspicion. If the patient is adolescent when first tested, the early stages of learning to read belong to the dimly remembered past, and it is often not clear whether the poor speller had originally been a late reader.

The suggestion that all persons notorious for their bad spelling are true dyslexia-variants cannot, however, be maintained. That is to say, some bad spellers are not, and never have been, dyslexic, and do not belong to a family where there are members with developmental dyslexia. How many cases of this kind with no link with poor reading is not yet known.

Sometimes a dyslexia-variant appears in a far more complicated guise, as, for example, in the following case:

"*Female, married, aged 41 years, was referred by her family doctor because of her inveterate difficulty with simple arithmetical calculations. The patient had never succeeded in learning her multiplication tables at school and she could not count up to 100. As an adult she contrived to conceal her predicament by memorising those products of multiplication which are in common use. An incorrigible confusion as to lateral dimensions also made it difficult for her to read a map, and it was often far from easy for her to find her way through familiar streets. As she put it, 'I orientate myself by the sun like a sailor at sea'.*
She had been late in learning to write, and had never attained competency in this art. Even when adult she found it burdensome to keep up her corres-

pondence. She insisted on using one particular fountain pen and none other. When writing even an informal letter to a close relative she had to make preliminary pencil headings, followed by a rough draft before her final version. She was also aware of disordered coordination. It was long before she learned to catch a ball successfully, and it was some years before she managed to ride a bicycle. She was never able to swim because she could not synchronize her breathing with the movements of her arms. She was quite a big girl before she could tie her shoe-laces. There was difficulty in acquiring techniques of dressmaking and even plain sewing, and she never mastered the ability to knit.

She was also very late in learning to tell the time, and the 24-hour clock was still beyond her powers of comprehension. She found driving a car difficult, and she had failed at least one driving test. She was unsuccessful in sight-reading music notation, on which account she gave up piano lessons. Although she had a good singing voice she reluctantly had to leave a choral society for she could not follow the music scores. She tried to learn to type, but eventually abandoned the attempt for she could not memorise the layout of the keyboard. When trying to cook a meal she would get into a hopeless muddle.

Jigsaw puzzles always proved most difficult, and she sorted the pieces according to colour rather than shape. On the other hand the patient learned to read early, and she soon began to read a great deal and with enjoyment. She was also an accurate speller until two years earlier when it had begun to deteriorate. She found she had to rely a good deal on a dictionary, although had no difficulty in looking up a word. Indeed she was employed for a time by the Post Office on Telephone Directory Enquiries.

All the other foregoing problems had been present for as long as she could remember. However, her son's serious illness two years earlier had worried her so much that all her disabilities worsened."

Such a complicated assembly of unusual cognitive troubles raises questions as to causation. The picture is certainly an "organic" one, and is not the expression of any neurosis. The symptoms might well have been ascribed to a structural lesion of the brain, particularly the parietal region. But the symptoms were not recent, and there was no evidence of long-standing brain-damage.

If one interprets correctly the word "dyslexia" as "difficulty with coping with words", then one can, without any affront to etymology and without resort to Procrustean thinking, include the notion of variants, incomplete exemplars, equivalents, or *formes frustes*, and even such a complex case as described above.

Another possible dyslexia-equivalent and a commoner, less elaborate one, may present itself in the guise of atrocious, barely legible handwriting, coupled with a mild degree of spelling-disability and unorthodox punctuation. The degree of distorted penmanship cannot be dismissed as the product of inherent clumsiness or lack of manual dexterity or tremulous hands. The magnitude of the difficulty presents a real handicap to the student, for the script may be unacceptable to examiners faced with the candidate's barely decipherable written work. Usually in these cases there has been no delay in learning to read, and no impairment in the speed or accuracy of reading. Should such an untidy writer belong to a family in which undoubted cases of developmental dyslexia have occurred, then the possibility of a dyslexia-variant seriously arises.

This type of *forme fruste* is common enough for examples to be quoted readily. Its frequency is shown by the fact that within a random test-period of 55 days, during which 44 new putative cases of developmental dyslexia were seen, four belonged to this particular type of dyslexia-variant. These are briefly quoted:

"*Male, aged 11·10 years, though of Polish ancestry, had been brought up as an Anglo-French bilingual. He learned to read early but his spelling was erratic in both of the languages which he could read and speak so well. Though he read for pleasure, he tended to choose books of a rather immature type. He was relatively slow in copying a text placed before him whether it were in English or in French. (G.U.S., 2·05 English, 1·95 French; normal 3). His spelling age in English was 9·06; unfortunately no scale of attainment in the French language was available at the time, but he was obviously more accurate in that language. The patient's handwriting was neat, small, and slightly recursive. There was a clear-cut family history of developmental dyslexia, and his brother, who undoubtedly had the problem, had also been seen and tested.*"

"*Male, aged 12·06 years, belonged to a family in which cases of reading and spelling disability were known. This boy, however, whose I.Q. was 120, read far beyond the 14-year level. His spelling age, on the other hand, was only 8. He wrote with painful slowness (G.U.S. 0·99; normal 3), and the resulting script was barely intelligible.*"

"*Male, aged 10·02, whose sister was a developmental dyslexic, was described as an avid reader especially of comics. His reading age proved to be 12·09, but his spelling age was less than 9. Essay-writing was particularly difficult for him to master, and his handwriting was grossly ill-formed, the individual characters being unusually large. He copied slowly (G.U.S. 1·13). Psychometric assessment revealed the boy to have a full-scale I.Q. of 127.*"

"*A left-handed boy of 8·11 years had been late in learning to read, but his present reading age was 13·06; he spelled, however, at an 8.06 year level. At home he was badly behaved, but not at school. His handwriting was ill-formed, being large and sprawling, and he was slow in copying. (G.U.S. 1·3).*"

Three more examples may be quoted which also fall within the category of dyslexia-equivalent.

"*Male, aged 10·03, of good intelligence and reading ability, was referred because of his appalling handwriting. The fault comprised more than an assemblage of ill-constructed letters with an overall untidiness; in addition, his compositions revealed a paucity of ideas, mistakes in syntax, omission of words, and capricious punctuation. In his writing, upper case and lower case letters were hopelessly jumbled. Testing with a stopwatch demonstrated that the act of writing—whether spontaneously, to dictation, or copying— was carried out slowly. His reading age was 13·06 and his spelling age 9·06. A definite history of developmental dyslexia was present on the paternal side of the family, together with a strong incidence of sinistrality on the maternal side.*"

"*Female, highly intelligent, of Italian stock. Her age was 12·04 and her reading age 12·0 She had always experienced difficulty in learning Latin and, to a lesser extent, French. In the latter language her spelling was even more erratic than in English, though it could not be assessed precisely. She found it hard to express her ideas on paper with facility and speed, and she had abandoned piano lessons on account of persistent difficulty in sight-reading a musical score. Her handwriting was outstandingly neat and graceful, but was executed slowly. (G.U.S. 1·51, i.e. just over half the expected figure). This girl had one brother and five sisters older than herself; all were poor spellers, as was her mother. The disability of the other children had, however, improved over the years, and from an academic standpoint they had all acquitted themselves with brilliance.*"

Perhaps one of the most striking cases of a dyslexia-variant was examined in 1941 and published in 1942. It concerned an intelligent officer-cadet in the Royal Navy who was found to be incapable of learning Morse telegraphy. Details of the case are as follows:

He was 21 years of age, with a very distinguished Naval background. There was no family history of any similar defects; nor of left-handedness, nor stammering. He attended a secondary school where his record, though never brilliant, was average. His attainments were patchy: he was ahead of his classmates in chemistry and mathematics. He fared best at geometry, for which he won a prize. English and French were easily his worst subjects, especially the latter. His difficulty did not concern grammar, only spelling. He was able to read normally, but is is uncertain whether he learned this accomplishment early or late. He left school at 15½ in Standard IV, at the same age as the other boys, in order to enter the Royal Navy. He went to H.M.S. "St. Vincent" where he was immediately relegated to the Superior Grade. After a year he passed on to H.M.S. "Iron Duke" for further training, and then served in H.M.S. "Courageous" for 2½ years. Afterwards he was appointed to H.M.S. "Dunedin", leaving to take a course ashore in order to qualify for advancement to Leading Torpedoman. These studies were interrupted when he was recommended for a special promotion course at H.M.S. "St. Vincent", with the object of passing from the lower to the quarterdeck. Confidential reports from his various Captains had hitherto marked him out as above average in intelligence, quickness and keenness. It was during the cadet-course that two main defects came to light, sufficiently severe and unusual to warrant medical referral. Briefly, his instructors found that whereas he was adequate at all other subjects he made grotesque spelling mistakes, and was quite unable to learn Morse signalling. The report of one of his officer-instructors read:

"He is so anxious to prove himself keen that he trips over himself. He is extremely well-mannered and polite and outwardly humble about his short-comings. He is smart in appearance, has an excellent bearing and speaks well. If integrity of character, loyalty and enthusiasm only were necessary, he would be a commissioned officer; but his appalling lack of intelligence where clear and rapid thought are required—practical navigation, etc.— quite rules out that possibility. He is an enigma. Undoubtedly keen and anxious to follow in the footsteps of his distinguished relatives, he shows knowledge and commonsense in matters of seamanship. Yet in class he visibly cracks during a prolonged period of instruction and seems to lack the mental stamina required for lengthy concentration. He becomes dull and sleepy. When asked a question that requires logical thinking or is at all off the beaten track, his mind becomes a chaos of disordered thoughts, and his attempts at an answer are incoherently expressed and often rank nonsense. His con-fusion of thought has been manifest most particularly in his spelling, and in his reading of the Morse code made on buzzer or lamp. His spelling mis-takes are not the usual ones of a normally bad speller. They are unique in that they consist of syllables transposed in a word or missed out altogether. Small words are often omitted and longer ones are deprived of their final letter. When reading the Morse code, even after eight months' daily practice, he cannot sort out the dots and dashes unless it is made very slowly".

At the end of his course he was recommended, not for a commission, but for advancement to the rank of Warrant Officer. He was transferred at this stage to a Naval hospital for fuller investigation. Some of the points in the instructor's report were substantiated though his comments upon general intellectual defects were not. At mental arithmetic he excelled and accurately substracted seven serially from 100 in 40 seconds. He could repeat nine digits forwards and at least eight digits backwards. His responses to tests of constructive thought were superior. Asked the difference between "character" and "reputation" he at once replied: "The character of a person is the educated instincts of that person; reputation is the opinion others have of him". On the revised Standford-Binet scale he showed a superior grade of intelligence. Tests for constructional apraxia were carried out without error. He was not altogether accurate in his estimation of distances, though the defect was in no way striking. Numerous and repeated tests clearly demonstrated that there was no evidence of spatial disorientation. (This point is important in view of the fact that the instructor had mentioned a tendency for him to confuse port and starboard while at the wheel.) No impairment was found when he read printed or written matter, whether silently or aloud.

Neurological and physical examination was negative, except for three types of disability, namely:

(1) Difficulty in spelling. This took the form of rather unusual errors. They were outstanding in frequency even when compared with the common mistakes of his contemporaries. A study of the "journal" which he maintained each day showed that he often omitted letters or groups of letters. He would at times reverse syllables or diphthongs, e.g. he might write BRITIAN for BRITAIN. As a rule he could not correct the mistakes when they were pointed out to him, and usually he did not recognise that the word had been mis-spelled. It had been reported that on occasions he made similar reversals in speech, when excited. Thus, when he wanted to say "*writhing* in pain" he came out with "*withering* in pain". This was, however, probably an isolated occurrence, and no spoonerisms or reversals of this sort were ever noticed in hospital.

(2) *Defects in signalling.* He showed himself efficient at semaphore and at interpreting hoists of signal-flags. He had always had considerable difficulty with Morse signals, especially in receiving messages. Although he had originally memorized the Morse alphabet within twenty minutes, he never became able to decode Morse signals with ease or rapidity despite long practice. When he was tested with flashing lights, these defects were well demonstrated. He was able to transmit quite accurately, though slowly. When, however, he tried to interpret a message which someone else was sending with an Aldis flash lamp, he failed utterly. He

explained his difficulty by saying that he was unable to distinguish between a dot and a dash, and that one symbol seemed to run into the next especially if the signals were given rapidly. There was no difficulty in decoding a small group of dashes and dots representing a letter of the alphabet, once he had read them clearly. When tested with a buzzer the same problem seemed to be apparent. This form of signalling was of course comparatively unfamiliar to him, as he had been taught signalling by way of a flash-lamp. He obviously found great difficulty in interpreting the sounds in terms of dots and he made far more errors than any normal control subject who was ignorant of Morse signalling. At times he was apt to omit dashes or dots from the middle or end of a signal, thus reading: —· · ·— as —· ·—; or — — — — as — — .

(3) *Defects in ciphering.* It was discovered that despite his skill at mental arithmetic, and his good visual memory, he made odd mistakes when instructed to write down on paper numbers which were dictated to him. Thus, when told to write "five million four hundred thousand and two" he put down 5,40002. "Three million, four hundred and five" was written as 30,4005. These mistakes he seemed not to recognise; nor could he correct them when they were pointed out.

In summary, then, it is suggested that developmental dyslexia does not always appear in a complete form, but that one or two of its constituent features can sometimes be seen in isolation. Thus, the patient may present as a case of extremely poor spelling; or bad handwriting to an extraordinary degree; in great confusion of lateral dimensions; in an inability of a musician to sight-read; and even, in special circumstances, incapacity to learn Morse. When such patients come from a family with one or more members with true developmental dyslexia, the diagnosis of a dyslexia-variant is likely; nonetheless without such a family history atypical cases certainly occur. To say this does not for one moment detract from the concept of developmental dyslexia as a definite organic neurological syndrome. There are many examples in medicine where a well-defined heredo-familial entity shows "pleotropic" characteristics, with some members exhibiting an incomplete, atypical, or a distorted version of the conventional clinical picture. Von Recklinghausen's neurofibromatosis, dystrophia myotonica, as well as the commonplace migraine, immediately come to mind. Epilepsy is an obvious example of a medical syndrome which, as is well known, may present itself in many guises other than repeated convulsive seizures. An axiom in neurology, first promulgated nearly a hundred years ago by Féré, was that there are as many epilepsies as epileptics. Every neurologist knows that no two cases of epilepsy, or for that matter of migraine, aphasia, multiple sclerosis or Parkinson's disease, are identical. The clinical findings are as personal as finger-prints. Experience also shows that no two dyslexics are wholly alike, but that does not deter one from recognising the picture and making a diagnosis of developmental dyslexia, any more than it does in a case of multiple sclerosis.

Apart from the subject of dyslexia-variants, the possibility of different clinical types of developmental dyslexia also comes up for discussion. Sometimes at the diagnostic interview, though more often during the course of remedial treatment, it may become evident that different perceptual problems, which interfere with the learning-processes, are entailed in different patients. To state that sub-types may occur in no way weakens the conception of developmental dyslexia as a specific entity.

Using the simplest possible terms, it can be said that many authorities on developmental dyslexia recognise two main types, namely auditory and visual. Ingram (1970) expanded this basic dichotomy and described an audiophonic, a visuospatial and a mixed variety (to which most of his patients seemed to belong). Boder (1971, 1973) has been one of the strongest advocates of recognisable types. Her terminology sounds formidable, for she has spoken of (1) a dysphonetic dyslexia; (2) a dyseidetic dyslexia (the Gestalt blind); and (3) mixed dysphonetic-dyseidetic types. Zangwill's three-fold classification is less convincing, for he leans not so much upon visual versus auditory types, but brings in the factor of imperfect cerebral laterality. He does not exclude from his series those children with minimal brain-dysfunction.

It is not always possible to make a distinction during a diagnostic interview, even though the remedial teacher may subsequently require to tailor or adapt her technique and to choose one approach rather than another.

It is interesting that S. Naidoo (1972) in her analysis of 98 boys retarded in reading and spelling investigated and treated at the former Word-Blind Centre, did not support the existence of clearly defined subgroups of dyslexia.

In '*The Dyslexic Child*" (1970) the question of possible sub-types was discussed but the conclusion was made that their isolation and evaluation was still a project for further inquiry rather than immediate acceptance. There does not seem to be any reason at present to change that opinion.

Chapter Ten

Arithmetical ability and dyslexia

"Calculation was formerly regarded as a particular ability of the merchant. Not until the eighteenth century, when children learned tables by heart at school, did arithmetic become a common ability . . . Thus calculation is not a primary or biological human capacity, but one which bears in its practical realization the stamp of our cultural configuration".

F. Grewel, 1952

Most dyslexics, whatever their age, seem to acquit themselves better at numeracy than at reading, writing and spelling. Even the highest peaks of mathematics have been scaled by graduates well-known as ex-dyslexics. Einstein is often quoted as a case in point, though the evidence for his being a true case of developmental dyslexia is slight. But he was certainly an indifferent scholar in his boyhood, and with his extremely high intelligence, this discrepancy in itself is suggestive.

It may be asked why numeracy should be less of a burden to dyslexics than the manipulation of words. First, there are more letters than digits, and they are more uniform in pattern. Furthermore, letters are far more abstract than numerals. In isolation a letter represents nothing substantial; a numeral, however, is meaningful in itself. Thus to a child the letter *M* is but one item out of a puzzling and considerable alphabet, while the sign *3* means just what it says, for it is a precise measurement of quantity. It is an index in mensuration. This distinction between abstract letters and concrete numbers is noticeable in Arabic—a complex language-system where the letter-symbols are read from right to left, changing their form according to the place they occupy within a word. Numerals are easier. Not only are they rigidly fixed in shape, but they proceed conspicuously from left to right, and are not joined together.

Although letters in isolation are more abstract than single digits, this does not apply to combinations of letters making up a word that is easily read and comprehended. Thus C, T, A standing alone do not mean much, but in appropriate conjunction, e.g. CAT, they are tangible, understandable, and not difficult. A grouping of three numerals, however, say 524, may be less obvious. It is believed that intelligibility as well as memory is greater for a long series of letters than of numbers. For example, the 14 letters which go to make up the word "transformation" are easier to hoist in, read aloud, comprehend and recall than a numerical series of similar length, e.g. 59677302910483. However, the group of letters in question would be harder if, as a cluster they were both unreadable and senseless, e.g. ZFGKOWVWLZCM-TT; and the 14-long numeral would become less obscure if it were broken up into thousands, millions and billions—59, 677, 302, 910, 483.

It could be argued that the dyslexic's relatively better performance with numeracy than with literacy may suffer if he is confronted early in his school-days with the Fletcher system of arithmetic, which makes use of letters and words as substitutes for figures.

We have reason to believe that from an evolutionary standpoint, our manner of calculation depends upon the fact that man is endowed with ten fingers. According to Aristotle, this is the origin of the decimal system. Nothing could be more material. The Romans used the word *digitum* to stand for either a finger or a number. The upraised fingers of one hand, used in a numerical sense, were symbolised by "V". "Four" was shown as "IV" or "hand minus one finger"; and "six" as "VI", or "hand plus one". If *homo sapiens* had happened to be furnished with six fingers, our modern decimal system would probably have never developed. An alternative system would have come about, and doubtless a more complicated one.

It must be realised, however, that some dyslectic children experience obstacles in the manipulation of numbers. Most are relatively late in learning to tell the time, an accomplishment which in Great Britain is widely expected to be achieved at about seven years of age. This is so despite the haphazard way children may pick it up from their parents or older children. As standard clock-faces gradually give way to digital dials, the practice of telling the time might be acquired at some age other than seven, and in the case of dyslexics the rapid transfer from one system to another may prove difficult. At an early age a child's uncertainty is shown when he draws a clock-face from memory. Young dyslexics usually demonstrate this confusion well. Individual numerals may be rotated. He may fail to set out the figures accurately on the dial within the rim of the circumference. Very occasionally the numbers are written in an anti-clockwise fashion. Dyslectic children usually interpret correctly a trick picture of a clock which has been deliberately drawn with the numbers the wrong way round, but this is perhaps an index of innate intelligence rather than of numeracy.

The other common difficulty with numbers experienced by dyslexics entails the memorising of the multiplication tables, and their ready recall. In part at least, this symptom is probably a mirror of the dyslexic's almost universal difficulty in sequential thinking or arranging things and ideas in the correct order. To be successful with his multiplication tables, a child must have an accessible visual memory and recall, something which is beyond the capabilities of most young dyslexics. These endowments can often be established by one of the subtests of that much favoured psychometric tool, the WISC (Wechsler Intelligence Scale for Children).

Another arithmetical impediment common in dyslexics results from their right-left confusion. Not only may he rotate a number so that it faces the wrong way, but he may also reverse two-digit figures, putting down 21 instead of 12. Or, as a kind of compromise, when asked to write "12" he may start with the "2" and then write the "1" on its left. The result is correct in appearance, but the manner of performance is unorthodox. These errors may also occur in figures of more than two digits.

The English-speaking dyslectic child eventually masters the fact that in order to constitute words, letters must be scanned from left to right. So it is with numerals, for 150,273 is pronounced "one hundred and fifty thousand, two hundred and seventy three'. But, the dyslexic may run into temporary difficulties with numerals when he begins to manipulate them. Addition, subtraction and multiplication are typically carried out from right to left, and for a time this difference may cause problems. Sexton has described a case of an educated ex-dyslectic 'teenager who, although good at trigonometry, occasionally made slips as when he wrote down the log of the denominator as ·3054 instead of ·4503. In languages other than English peculiar difficulties may arise because of the unorthodox way numbers are read aloud. Although a Frenchman will say 42 (*quarante-deux*) he will speak of 4-twenties and nine for 89 (*quatre vingts neuf*). In the Basque language, numerals are based upon a ventigesimal system, 40, 60 and 80 being respectively spoken of as two score (*hogoi*), three score (*hiruten hogoi*), and four score (*lauretan hogoi*). Danish is similar, in that 60 is called three-twenties (*tresindstyre*). A German, on the other hand, will say 16 and 18 (*sechszehn, achtzehn*) but always 9 and 20 (*neun und zwanzig*), 8 and 80 (*acht und achtzehn*) for 29 and 88, respectively.

Another hazard commonly comes to light on appropriate testing. Just as the developmental dyslexic finds it hard to spell a word dictated to him, so he also perpetrates errors when "spelling" numbers. These usually concern the nought or zero, as well as the proper placement of commas. Thus, a dyslectic schoolboy may be perplexed when asked to write twenty thousand and two, or one million and one, offering "2020", "220", "2,20", "2,020"; or "10,001", "100,01", "1,0,001".

As a rule these hindrancies are not severe enough to prevent him from coping with arithmetic, and, later, with simple mathematics adequately and even well. Often a dyslexic says this is a subject which he enjoys, and it helps him to compensate for his poor showing at tasks entailing literacy.

As the subject of mathematics becomes more intricate later in the school curriculum, new problems arise. Written questions now tend to be lengthy and complicated. Reading with complete accuracy is essential, otherwise the answers will be hopelessly wrong. In an examination, meticulous reading and re-reading of the question consumes valuable time, but the task is all-important and examiners should be alerted to the candidate's predicament. In a schoolboy with developmental dyslexia, the arithmetical difficulties ordinarily go deeper.

Sexton (1963) has quoted two typical examples of mathematical problems where a dyslexic, by skipping a simple preposition, missed the complete significance of the question and perpetrated gross errors in interpretation. In the first example, which read "*what will be the volume of gas if the pressure is reduced to 18 lbs. per square inch*", all four dyslexics who tackled the question omitted to notice the word "to". They tried to answer the question as though it read "*if the pressure is reduced 18 pounds per square inch*". In the second instance, "*the product of two consecutive odd integers is 50 less than the square of the greater*", the pupil skipped the word "than" and proceeded to tackle *"the product of two consecutive odd integers is 50 less the square of the greater"*.

Unfortunately, some writers have used the word "dyscalculia" when referring to a dyslexic's difficulty with arithmetic. A neurologist uses this term to describe the loss resulting from acquired brain-disease of the faculty of reckoning and all other aspects of numerical thinking.

Confusion between such contrasting notions as: more than/less than; larger/smaller; add/subtract; multiply/divide; and the notions of fractions, percentages, square roots, and the science of trigonometry, vanish early in cases of acquired dyscalculia.

In a dyslexic, it must be remembered, a good knowledge of mathematics entails the embodiment of a formidable number of technical terms which in themselves may prove a stumbling block to a dyslexic whose overall vocabulary is limited. Such expressions as "co-efficient", "dividend", "quotient", "subtrahend", "binominal", "perimeter" may also be a serious hindrance for even an arithmetically-minded dyslexic. It is not the mathematical concept that is difficult, but the correct reading of the terms.

Lack of number-sense rarely occurs in children with developmental dyslexia, though of course it does so in cases of secondary dyslexia. In other words, a combination of severe reading problems with difficulty in differentiating between such concepts as more than/less than; smaller/larger; higher/lower, half/twice, should always raise the suspicion of either low intelligence or else minimal brain-dysfunction.

In the literature on dyslexia, and more particularly on "specific learning disabilities", references are occasionally made to "congenital dyscalculia". Though not a topic germane to this book, it deserves a brief mention, if only because, if it exists, it may represent yet another instance of a localised maturational lag. If so, it could conceivably be present in association with a developmental dyslexia, resulting in an inborn delay in both literacy and numeracy.

Congenital dyscalculia, if it exists, must be rare. What is implied is a medley of defects comparable with those which follow certain forms of disease of the adult brain. These would extend beyond a mere hesitancy in reckoning, whether on paper or as a mental operation, and include an upset in the fundamental conceptions of number-sense.

Chapter Eleven

"Soft" neurological signs: what does it mean?

" There were men of pith and thew
Whom the city never called
Scarce could read or hold a quill,
But built the barn, the forge, the mill".

Edmund Blunden

Writers dealing with the dyslexias, particularly in the United States, often refer to "soft neurological signs" but without clearly defining the term. Who was first responsible for the expression is uncertain. Presumably what is implied is that collection of subtle neurological signs which fails to be uncovered on ordinary, that is, routine medical examination. The inference is that an "extended" or more exacting scrutiny of nervous function would uncover minimal defects and deviations in children with specific learning disorders, and are hence of diagnostic value.

Rabinovitch, for example, set out a number of deficits which might come to light in dyslexics as the result of what he called an "expanded neurological examination". They included (1) disorders of spatial thought; (2) impaired notions of time; (3) inconsistent or mixed cerebral dominance; (4) disorders of articulate speech; (5) anomalies of motility; and (6) poor figure-background discrimination. He considered that the last two were especially important in very young subjects.

Earlier in this book it was mentioned that some of the neurological manifestations of both secondary as well as developmental dyslexics, are reminiscent of the signs of acquired disease of the parietal or parieto-occipital lobes in an adult's brain. One author has claimed that dyslectic children cannot name colours, or are conspicuously late in learning to do so. One must not conclude, however, that, when present in the developing child all the various quasiparietal signs connote a structural lesion.

Some of the "soft" signs have already been described and need merely to be recapitulated. These include delay in learning to tell the time: right-left confusion leading to rotations and reversals in writing and persisting well into childhood. Clumsiness and imperfect coordination are regarded by some as "soft" signs, a topic which was discussed more fully in Chapter 6, where doubt was expressed as to their place in the context of developmental dyslexia.

Another "soft" sign comprises the "postural reflexes" evoked by turning the child's head to one side and then the other, the arms being outstretched and the eyelids closed. A positive response is shown by the child unconsciously deviating his arms to the side towards which the head is turned.

Another "soft" sign, already mentioned, consists in "synkinesia". This is a technical term applied to the phenomenon whereby forceful or intricate actions deliberately carried out with one hand, are faintly but unwittingly "mirrored" by small-range similar movements in the other hand.

Some writers have looked upon certain other clinical findings as "soft" signs. These include a hesitancy on the part of the child when he is asked to name or point to individual fingers; inability to catch a ball, to skip or to hop; to manipulate with dexterity constructional toys such as Lego; to draw; to imitate a tapped-out rhythm; to reproduce geometrical shapes from memory after they have been briefly displayed and then withdrawn (Benton's test); difficulties in articulate speech; hyperactivity; gross limitation of the span of attention; evidence of infirm cerebral dominance; and "motor impersistence" or failure to maintain adequately a particular movement. From the literature it is evident that the last named sign was originally described as an index of cerebral damage.

This medley of clinical signs and symptoms is diverse in nature, and obviously represents different levels of importance and frequency. Some of these signs are highly suggestive of a "secondary" dyslexia. Others, it is true, may be met with in some cases of developmental dyslexia, though in that case the age of the child is all-important as to whether one might expect to find some of them on examination.

Those "soft" signs which may be apparent in cases diagnosed as developmental dyslexia comprise: delay in learning to read a clock; right-left confusion; postural reflexes; synkinesia; possibly impaired ability to reproduce rhythms; and mild degrees of inattention. Postural reflexes and synkinesia are, of course, normal findings in very young children, but they should disappear by the age of about six years. In developmental dyslexics they may persist rather longer, perhaps another 12 or 18 months. Should they still be demonstrable after the age of eight, then the suspicion that the case is one of "secondary" dyslexia becomes considerable. As already stated, it has been claimed by one author that dyslectic children cannot name colours, or else are late in doing so. In our series of more than two thousand true cases of developmental dyslexia, this symptom has not yet been demonstrated although the patients were specifically tested.

Some other 'soft" signs are purely coincidental and have no bearing upon the diagnosis of developmental dyslexia. When they are present they are nothing more than "epiphenomena". Here belong the milder states of overactivity up to the age of puberty; inability to concentrate except upon tasks which are pleasurable; and such speech-disorders as delayed talking and indistinct articulation.

The symptom of hyperactivity, sometimes amounting to what is called the "syndrome of the hyperkinetic child", should not be over-emphasised in the context of developmental dyslexia. One says this advisedly, because in the U.S.A. there has been a vogue for treating poor readers with drugs directed towards the control of hyperkinesis. Oddly enough, these drugs are not tranquillisers but stimulants, and one cannot overstress the fact that they are not only useless for dyslexics, but potentially dangerous. Fortunately, in Great Britain they cannot be legally dispensed and are, therefore, unavailable here even on prescription.

The spontaneous drawings of a dyslexic are occasionally odd, even outlandish. They may be far too small in size; ill-formed; and not much more than a scribble. In itself poor drawing means little from a diagnostic point of view. Perhaps the child has no aptitude, and will never draw well; many do not. Perhaps his spatial orientation is uncertain. Maybe poor drawing by a child is just another mark of cerebral immaturity which eventually will right itself. Gratuitous introduction of detail in a drawing, however odd, betrays imagination. Very occasionally a child will draw a landscape, or a bicycle from an unorthodox angle, that is to say, viewed from above instead of from the side, or as seen from the front or the back. On the other hand, some developmental dyslexics show skill not only in drawing but also in the use of colour as well as in clay-modelling, metal-work and pottery. There is no rule about artistic achievement in dyslexics.

Right-left confusion is almost universal in developmental dyslexics. Though it tends to improve as the child grows older, it may continue to some extent well into adulthood, or even be life-long.

"Soft" neurological signs are, therefore, not as significant in the diagnosis of developmental dyslexia as they are in cases of secondary dyslexia. We probably still need more knowledge of developmental behaviour in control subjects (that is, non-dyslexics), so that we can state with greater confidence the age at which certain hallmarks of immaturity should normally have been obliterated. At the same time, the presence of what we might call acceptable soft signs are of some value in young children, for they give the lie to the contention that developmental dyslexia is a condition which can be diagnosed only by a process of elimination.

Chapter Twelve

The nature of developmental dyslexia: summing-up

"4th September
Dear Sir,
At the school I was at I did not like it at all because of the boys and the
teachers and because they know that they know that am not strong so they
fight me and I cannot do the work and they laugh at me and I get a pain in
my stomach and I get ill and I would like to go to a school where there are
boys like me and I do not mind if it is a boarding school at all. and they
make me read in front of boys and I perspire and the same thing happened
at the other three schools and am last in all the sports except swimming
*   from*
*   Christopher."*

'Well, the next part was books. I suddenly, you know, discovered what
they were. I'd read things before, of course, but it had always been to fill in
time while I was waiting for something else, and now I suddenly saw them
differently, in rows and rows and rows, each with a secret in it like a nut,
and I cracked them and ate them and had the greatest fun. Then I began to
think that I was awfully clever and that I would write great books
myself . . ."   *Hugh Walpole: Maradick at Forty.*

"Forty years long was I grieved with this generation, and said: it is a
people that do err in their heart, for they have not known my ways."
                                                                    Venite

Accepting the concept of a specific syndrome of poor readers,
writers and spellers who also have a problem expressing themselves
easily or fluently on paper, the most favoured hypothesis today as
to the cause of developmental dyslexia is *a delay in the maturation of*
those parts of the brain which are concerned with reading-skills. No crude
structural lesion of the brain is visualized, and it is likely that if a
pathologist were to make an autopsy he would not be able to

detect any physical abnormality on either naked-eye or micro-scopical examination of the brain. In other words, the fault is one of function and not of structure.

The manifold activities subserved by the brain such as move-ment, perception, vision, memory, thinking, understanding, cogitation, language, are not all present at birth. They gradually develop as the infant grows. Moreover these functions do not mature synchronously, any more than all the flowers in a garden suddenly burst into bloom on a particular date. Like blossoms, some functions come into being early, others late; most are intermediate as to their time of flowering.

Early this century, a German neuro-anatomist, Paul Flechsig, studied the relative rate of maturation of various areas of the brain. His technique was to look for the first signs of "myelina-tion"; that is to say, the moment when the intracerebral nerve-fibres become invested with their insulating sheaths which are composed of a fatty-like substance known as myelin. From his careful researches Flechsig was able to ascertain that in some areas of the brain myelination appears early, in others it is later, and here and there later still. From these data he was able to con-struct an interesting brain-map. Roughly speaking, the regions of the brain which myelinate last are those which we tie up with the most highly evolved functions, that is, those that are associated with the uppermost activities of the nervous system. These are the areas which are specific for man not even appearing in the highest primates. Among them reside the more complicated processes of learning.

Flechsig's evidence as to the selective maturation of regions of the brain was, be it noted, anatomical in nature, for it involved the presence or absence of a particular intracerebral tissue-structure. To a large extent, furthermore, myelination correlates with nervous function.

Many scientists believe, however, that function does not depend exclusively upon whether or not the nerve-fibres are insulated by fatty sheaths. Myelin might be there but without all of the nerve-cells being yet fully operative. Function thus lies dormant for an undue period, although the anatomical structure stands ready and expectant. There are precedents elsewhere in the human organ-ism. For example, the organs of speech are fully formed both in the brain and in the larynx even before the acquisition of that faculty. This applies to man as well as other primates. Why structure should precede function is an interesting topic, but inappropriate for discussion here.

However, conceivably the link is chemical, and one which precedes myelination, it being a transaction which lies within the territory of biological chemistry and might well be susceptible to delay because of some inherent and genetically determined process. Equally, the chemistry of myelin might be capable of stimulation by artificial means. Were that to happen, we should also be in possession of a method whereby the natural processes of learning might be artificially accelerated.

Quite apart from the chemistry of the myelin-sheaths investing the axonal processes of each nerve-cell, scientists are able to study the neuron itself with its complicated nuclear structure, as well as the complex means whereby adjacent and also remote cells communicate with each other.

Still thinking along purely structural lines we must remember the sheer complexity of the physical organ of mind. The human brain contains at least ten thousand million neurons or nerve-cells embodied within an elaborate supporting tissue of glial cells and their fibres. Each neuron is linked to one or more nerve-cells by a vast number of connecting nerve-fibres, so that cells do not act in isolation but operate within a far-flung organisation. When it comes to an elaborate intellectual cognitive activity such as learning, the complexity is almost beyond imagination. From a structural point of view, it is known that every nerve-cell is linked up with another by at least 10,000 fibrillary processes, in a fashion that is incredibly complex. The transmission of impulses from cell to cell is furthermore mediated by neurohumoral or chemical "transmitter substances". We already know of the existence of at least five such substances, and the total will surely turn out to be far greater than this. Already we are familiar with what takes place in the brain when one of these known chemical neurohumoral transmitters is lacking, and what happens when we deliberately replace it: that is, the loss of dopamine from certain nerve-cells of the brain in Parkinson's disease and its restoration by taking L-Dopa by mouth. If it were one day possible to demonstrate an inborn anomaly of a neurohumoral transmitter in the brain of a child with developmental dyslexia, then the possibility of replacing it pharmacologically becomes quite conceivable.

These remarks are, of course, purely speculative today, but they are not inherently improbable. Extensive biochemical research of the brain is fortunately under way all over the world, often with dramatic results, which may have a practical application as well as fundamental scientific value in connection with the processes of learning.

Summary

It is appropriate, in concluding this final chapter, to revert to some of the matters raised in Chapter 1, especially attacks upon the concept of dyslexia, as well as nomenclature. Most of the neglect of the problem 30 or 40 years ago was due to sheer unawareness by educationalists of the medical interest in cases of learning disability. As a matter of fact, some of those earlier critics have since become convinced supporters of the concept of developmental dyslexia.

For a long time critics have spoken of a "continuum" of badreaders but without leaving any niche for the small "specific" nub or core envisaged by neurologists. Professor Meredith, however, takes exception to the use of "continuum", and Professor Tropp, too, is critical. White Franklin (1972) has also written "the argument that children with specific dyslexia form part of a "continuum" of reading abilities is a concept already discarded by the more open-minded psychologists and should now be decently buried".

The objection was raised that no definition exists of dyslexia (or of developmental dyslexia), regardless of the fact that it was defined in 1942 by Skydsgaard, by Hermann (1956), by Eisenberg in 1966, and by many others. When attention was drawn to the fact that specific developmental dyslexia was also clearly defined by the World Federation of Neurology in 1968, a few writers demurred that this was not an "operational" definition. This objection has already been referred to in Chapter 1. Incidentally the expression "operational definition" had already been explicitly mentioned and given by Eisenberg in 1966, and it deserves quotation: "Operationally, specific reading disability may be defined as the failure to learn to read with normal proficiency despite conventional instruction, a culturally adequate home, proper motivation, intact senses, normal intelligence, and freedom from gross neurological defects."

The next objection was that the World Federation of Neurology's definition is one of mere elimination. This point has been raised from time to time. The critics added a rider to the effect that "if so" (i.e. diagnosis by exclusion) "the result is a council of despair, indeed". This throw-away comment is an emotive and meaningless one. As already said, many disorders are diagnosed by exclusion.

The phrase "despite conventional instruction" was then seized upon and the question asked whether it meant that dyslexia could not be diagnosed in a child taught by i.t.a. This is manifestly a *non sequitur*. "Conventional instruction" referred to attendance at school and the ministrations of trained teachers, and not to the precise techniques adopted for teaching a child to read. They queried "despite adequate intelligence" and asserted that this implies "that dyslexia cannot occur in children with below-average intelligence". Again this is wrong, as was clearly said in "The Dyslexic Child" (1970). Developmental dyslexia can occur in any child, whatever its intelligence quotient.

Again, "socio-cultural opportunity" implied to them that a child from a deprived background never suffers from developmental dyslexia. No such inference was made, because developmental dyslexia obviously can and does exist in such circumstances.

In 1975 Rutter and Yule asserted that "there has been a complete failure to show that the signs of dyslexia constitute any meaningful pattern" . . . that "up to now there is no evidence for the validity of a single special syndrome of dyslexia"; that "dyslexia remains a rather dubious hypothesis with very little evidence in support", and finally, "the concept of dyslexia (as usually proposed) remains a hypothesis for which evidence is so far lacking".

That there is no single "pathognomic" or specifically characteristic feature by which one can recognize the syndrome is quite true, and was emphasized in "The Dyslexic Child" (1970). But the same argument could be used for many disease-states in neurology and medicine—perhaps most.

Many who have criticised the concept of developmental dyslexia have been prepared to admit the existence of a group of children who, they say, are victims of "specific reading retardation" (S.R.R.). Is this entity the same as developmental dyslexia? The critics seem inconsistent or ambivalent on this score. Sometimes they seem to suggest that they are; at other times that they are not. If they allege, as did Rutter (1975), that S.R.R. is a syndrome which also includes (1) considerable arithmetical difficulties; (2) severe problems in spelling; (3) delay in the development or maturity of language power between 9 and 10 years; (4) incoordination; (5) motor impersistence; (6) right-left confusion; (7) possible difficulties in constructional tasks; (8) strong family history of reading difficulties; and (9) no association with sinistrality or mixed handedness, then obviously S.R.R. is not developmental dyslexia.

Professor Miles' rejoinder is that "as things are, they have set up an Aunt Sally, and, by knocking it down, have thereby given comfort to the forces of inertia and reaction" (1972).

Professor Rutter's article "The Concept of Dyslexia" (1969) contained many captious animadversions, and yet by an odd type of alchemy, his summary was in a much gentler vein. It can be quoted here, verbatim:

"There can be no doubt that the concept of 'dyslexia' has been most useful in highlighting the importance of these developmental neurological abnormalities. On the other hand there is nothing to suggest that "dyslexia" is a single condition distinguished by its purity and gravity. There may well be several 'dyslexias' which are due to different factors but which are united by the fact that each variety is due to some developmental neurological anomaly . . . In so far as the matter has been examined, the *prognosis and response to treatment of 'dyslexic' children does not seem to be very different from other children with reading retardation of equivalent severity.* Obviously the matter requires further research and the issue is far from settled, but perhaps one should question the assumption that 'dyslexic' children need a completely different form of teaching from that required by other children with severe reading retardation. No one method will ever be suitable for all children and whatever the diagnosis, the plan and treatment will have to be based on the nature and extent of the individual child's biological, social and psychological handicaps—not just on a diagnostic label".

The epigram "purity and gravity" was quoted from "Developmental Dyslexia", M. Critchley (1964), but the author had in fact made it clear that it was not original and had been said by someone else.

Nor should one allow to pass unchallenged, the sentence printed here in italics. A very considerable follow-up experience of dyslectic children who failed to make headway at school until specialized remedial therapy had been started shows that they then advanced. It is doubtful whether a comparable degree of betterment is achieved by children with other kinds of reading retardation.

Professor Vernon, originally a critic of the concept of developmental dyslexia, is now a supporter, though she has stated "They are often extremely resistant to remedial teaching". Mr. Yule, a critic of dyslexia and an advocate of the term specific reading retardation, has confessed (1975) "many parents will, however, be disappointed that we cannot go further and advise on what to do to help the children with S.R.R. As we all know, the literature on the effects of remedial reading teaching is far from helpful . . .".

Why these striking differences of opinion? It seems to turn upon the dissimilar experience of the academics and the practitioners. Long acquaintance with the problem leaves one in no doubt: the majority of cases of developmental dyslexia will respond to the prompt institution of intensive remediation at the hands of a teacher qualified in one of the special techniques of instruction. Do all dyslexics make good progress? Perhaps not. Some of those with direct responsibility for remediation have said in personal communications, that within the diagnosed cases of developmental dyslexia there may be a few who prove intractable to all forms of remedial help. Dr. Lucius Waites of Dallas in a personal discussion said that 5 per cent of all his cases of developmental dyslexics do not fare well. This figure is considerably higher than the estimate personally given by Mrs. Helen Arkell. An inquiry into the prognosis of all treated cases of developmental dyslexia would be an important project for research. Perhaps it might turn out that the intractable cases are those dyslectic children bereft of all five items of the "prognostic pentagon" mentioned earlier.

Probably the most tragic outcome of all this wordy controversy is that it gives some educational authorities an excuse for doing little or nothing to help the child with developmental dyslexia. The setting-up of the Tizard Committee was a great opportunity for directing the attention of teachers and educators to the existence of a group of non-achievers who could be helped if only more enthusiastic help were forthcoming, entailing the teaching of teachers, and the setting up of a corps of specialist remedial experts. As Miles put it "if you (i.e. the writers of the Tizard and of the Bullock Reports) were to say 'we recognise dyslexia as a problem, but we are doing nothing about it as we have not the money or the teachers', this would at least be honest; what seems to me manifestly absurd is to refuse to recognise dyslexia on the grounds that other children need help in other ways!"

And so things stand in 1977. Parents may, however, take heart in the knowledge that matters are steadily improving, though with painful slowness. The intervention of the Courts of Law and also of the Ombudsman have proved successful at times but such costly and tardy intervention should not be needed. Legal delays deprive the child of years of remedial help, so that it is even more difficult for him to catch up.

The protaganists and antagonists of dyslexia need their heads knocking together. If the antagonists will change their "specific reading retardation" to "specific *learning* retardation", they might accept a modified definition of "specific developmental dyslexia".

We agree that stylistically the World Federation of Neurology's definition of 1968 could be bettered and made simpler. In its place, the following longer definition is submitted: Developmental Dyslexia:

"*A learning-disability which initially shows itself by difficulty in learning to read, and later by erratic spelling and by lack of facility in manipulating written as opposed to spoken words. The condition is cognitive in essence, and usually genetically determined. It is not due to intellectual inadequacy or to lack of socio-cultural opportunity, or to faults in the technique of teaching, or to emotional factors, or to any known structural brain-defect. It probably represents a specific maturational defect which tends to lessen as the child grows older, and is capable of considerable improvement, especially when appropriate remedial help is afforded at the earliest opportunity*".

References

Agate, J. (1935), *Ego*, London: Hamish Hamilton.

Ajuriaguerra, J. (1960), *Psych. de l'enf.*, **3**, 609–718.

Bakker, D., Smink, T. and Reitsema, P. (1973), *Cortex*, **9**, 310–312.

Blanchard, P. (1936), *Ment. Hyg.*, **20**, 384–413.

Blanchard, P. (1946), *Psychoanal. Stud. Child.*, **2**, 163–188.

Boder, E. (1970), *J. Sch. Health.*, **40**, 289–290.
Developmental Dyslexia: prevailing diagnostic concepts and a new diagnostic approach from: *Progress in Learning Disabilities.* Ed. H. R. Myklebut. Vol. 2.

Bullock Report (1975), *A Language for Life*, H.M. Stationery Office, London.

Burt, C. (1946), *The Backward Child*, 2nd Edition, p. 166. London: ULP.

Carbonnell de Grampone (1974) *Acad. Ther.*, **9**, 5.
Quoted from Tarnopol, and Tarnopol, M. (1976) in: *Reading Disabilities: An International Perspective.* Univ. Park Press., Balt., Lond., Tokyo.

Chesni, Y. (1959), *Rev. neur.*, **101**, 576–582.

Claiborne, J. H. (1906), *J. Am. med. ass.*, **47**, 1813–1816.

Clark, M. M. (1957), *Left-Handedness. Laterality Characteristics and their Educational Implications.* London: ULP.

Cole, M. (1964), *Neurol.*, **14**, 968–970.

Crabtree, T. (1976), *Evening Standard*, 16 Feb.

Critchley, M. (1942), *J. Mount Sinai Hosp.* **9**, 363–375.

Critchley, M. (1953), *The Parietal Lobes*, London, Arnold.

Critchley, M. (1964), *Developmental Dyslexia*, Wm. Heinemann Books Ltd., London.

Critchley, M. (1966), *Brain*, **89**, 183–198.

Critchley, M. (1970), *The Dyslexic Child*, Wm. Heinemann Medical Books Ltd., London.

Critchley, M. (1963), Language and Communication, McGraw-Hill Book Co., N.Y. (paperback).

Darwin, C. (1872), *The Expression of the Emotions in Animals.* Murray, London.

Eisenberg, L. (1966), *Pediatrics*, **37**, 352.

Elliott and Needleman (1976), *Brain & Lang*, **3**, 339–349.

Faust, C. (1954), *Nervenartz*, **25**, 137.

Fildes, L. G. (1921), *Brain*, **44**, 286–307.

Flechsig, P. (1920), *Anatomic des menslichen Gehirns und Ruckemarks auf myelogenetischer Grundlage. Leipsig: Thieme.*

Ford, F. R. (1960), *Diseases of the Nervous System in infancy, childhood, & adolescence.* (4th Ed.) C. Thomas, Springfield, Ill.

Franklin, A., White (1972), *Dyslexia Review*, 7–9.

Frith, Uta (1976), *Trans. Brit. Assoc.*, **115** (quoted 'The Times' 4.9.76).

Gill, E. (1931), *An Essay on Typography.*

Goodman, K. S. (1970), "Reading, Process & Program", Urbana, Ill.

Gowers, W. (1902), *Lancet*, **i**, 1002–1007.

Gubbay, *et al* (1965), *Brain*, **88**, 295–312.

Gubbay (1973), *Proc. Australian Ass. Neur.*, **10**, 19–25.

Hallgren, B. (1950), *Acta. psych. neur. Suppl.* No. 65, 1–287.

Harrigan, J. E. (1976), *J. Learning Disabilities*, **9**, 74–80.

Harris, A. J. (1957), *J. Psychol.*, **44**, 283–294.

Hermann, K. and Norrie, E. (1958), *Psych. Neur.*, **136**, 59–73.

Hermann, K. (1959), *Reading Disability*, Copenhagen: Munsgaard.

Hinshelwood, J. (1898), *Lancet*, **i**, 422–425.

Hinshelwood, J. (1917), *Congenital Word-Blindness*, Lewis: London.

Huttenlocher, P. R. and Huttenlocher, J. (1973), *Neurol.*, **23**, 1107–1116.

Jacoby, H. J. (1939), *Analysis of Handwriting.*

Jansky, J. J. (1973), *Bull. Orton Soc.*, **23**, 78–79.

Jones, Daniel (1977), *My friend Dylan Thomas*: J. M. Dent and Sons Ltd.

Klein, E. (1949), "Psychoanalytic Study of the Child." N.Y. International Universities Press, III–IV, 369–390.

Kline, C. L. and Lee, N. (1971), *J. Spec. Educ.*, **6**, 9–26.

Kline, C. L. and Lee, N. (1969), *Bull. Orton Soc.*, **19**, 67–80.

Kuromaru, S. and Okada, S. 'On Developmental Dyslexia in Japan.' *Trans. 7 Internat. Congress Neurol.* Rome.

Langford, W. S., de Hirsch, K. and Jansky, J. J. (1962–65). *The Prediction of Reading, Writing and Spelling Disabilities in Children.* Report to the Health Research Council. City of N.Y.

Levy, J. and Reid, M. (1976), *Science,* **194**, 337.

Lorge, J. and Thorndike, E. L. (1959), *The Teacher's Word book of 30,000 words.* Bureau of Publ. Teachers' Coll., Columbia Univ., N.Y. 3rd impression.

McLeod, J. (1966), *Bull. Orton, Soc.*, **16**, 14–23.

Macmeeken, M. (1939), *Ocular Dominance in relation to Developmental Aphasia.* London: ULP.

Makita, K. (1968), *Am. J. Orthopsych.*, **38**, 599–614.

Masland, R. (1976), *Bull. Orton. Soc.*, **26**, 10–18.

Mayaruma, M. (1958), *Bull. Orton. Soc.*, **8**, 14–16.

Mehegan, C. C. and Dreifuss, F. E. (1972), *Neurol.*, **22**, 1105–1111.

Meredith, P. (1972), *Dyslexia Review*, 12–13.

Miles, T. R. (1972), *Dyslexia Review*, 11–12.

Miller, G. (1951), Language and Communication., McGraw-Hill Book Co., N.Y. (paperback, 1963).

Naidoo, S. (1972), *Specific Dyslexia*, London: Pitman.

Nazarova, L. K. (1952), *Soviet. Pedag.*, **6**.

Newton, M. with Ratcliff, C. (1974), *The Aston Index*: University of Aston, Birmingham.

Ogden, C. K. and Richards, J. (1923), *The Meaning of Meaning*, Harcourt, Bruce and Co., N.Y.

Orton, S. T. (1943), *Arch. ophth.*, **30**, 707–713.

Orton, S. T. (1943), *Arch. ophth.*, **14**, 581.

Pratt, R. T. C. and Warrington, E. K. (1972), *Brit. J. Psychiatr.*, **121**, 327–328.

Rabinovitch. R. D. (1956), *Research Publ. Assoc. Nerv. Ment. Dis. Research Approach to Reading*, **34**, 363–396. Retardation in *Res. Publ. Ass. Res. Nerv. Ment. Dis.*, **34**, 363–396.

Rawson, M. B. (1968), *Development Language Disability: Adult Accomplishments of Dyslexic Boys, Monogr. No. 2*. Hood Coll., Baltimore: Johns Hopkins Press.

Rozin, P., Poritzley, S. and Sotsky, R. (1971), *Science.*, **171**, 1264–1271.

Rutter, M. (1969), *Planning for Better Learning*. Ed. P. H. Wolff and R. MacKeith, London, 1969. In assoc. with Wm. Heinemann Medical Books Ltd., pp. 129–139.

Rutter, M. and Yule, W. (1975), *J. Child Psychol. Psychiatr.*, **16**, 181–197.

Satz. P. *et al.* (1975), *Bull. Orton. Soc.*, **69**, **91–110**.

Silberberg, N. E. and Silberberg, M. C. (1967), *Except. Child.*, **34**, **41**.

Sladen, B. K. (1970), *Bull. Orton. Soc.*, **20**, 30–40.

Sladen, B. K. (1972), *Bull. Orton. Soc.*, **22**, 41–53.

Skydsgaard (1942), *Den Konstitutionelle Dyslexi*: Copenhagen.

Subirana, A. (1969), *Handbook Clin. Neur.* Vol. 4: Amsterdam.

Subirana, A. (1952), *Schwz. Arch. Neur. Psych.*, **69**, 321–359.

Tizard Report (1972), H.M. Stationery Office, London.

Tower, D. M. (1973), *Bull. Orton. Soc.*, **23**, 78–89.

Tropp, A. (1972), *Dyslexia Review*, 9–10.

Tropp, A. (1974), ,, ,, 7–9.

Vernon, M. D. (1975), *Backwardness in Reading: A Study of its nature and origin*: Camb. Univ. Press.

Vernon, M. D. (1975), *Dyslexia Review*, 8–11.

Vernon, M. D. (1962), *B. J. Educ. Psychol.*, **32**, 143.

Wada, J. and Rasmussen, T. (1960), *J. Neurosurg.*, **17**, 266–282.

Walton, J., Ellis, E. and Court, S. D. M. (1952), *Brain.*, **85**, 603–612.

Warrington, E. K. and Pratt, R. T. C. (1973), *Neuropsychol.*, **11**, 423–428.

Yule, W. (1976) (Editorial), *Psychol. med.*, **6**, 165–167.

Yule, W. (1975), *Dyslexia Review*, 11–15.

Zangwill, O. (1960), *Central dominance and its relation to psychological function*, Edinburgh: Oliver and Boyd.

Zangwill, O. (1962), *Reading Disability*, (Edit. J. Money), Chap. 7, John
Hopkins Press, Baltimore.

Index